Current Clinical Strategies

Pediatrics 5-Minute Reviews

New AAP Guidelines

2001-2002 Edition

Karen Scruggs, MD

Michael T. Johnson, MD

Current Clinical Strategies Publishing

www.ccspublishing.com/ccs

Digital Book and Updates

The digital book and updates of this text can be downloaded via the Internet at the Current Clinical Strategies Publishing Web site: www.ccspublishing.com/ccs

Current Clinical Strategies Publishing
27071 Cabot Road
Laguna Hills, California 92653
Phone: 800-331-8227
Fax: 800-965-9420
info@ccspublishing.com
Internet: www.ccspublishing.com/ccs

Printed in USA   ISBN 1881528-98-7

Contents

Neonatology

Normal Newborn Care

I. **Prenatal pediatric visit**
   A. The prenatal pediatric visit usually takes place during the third trimester of the pregnancy. Maternal nutrition, the hazards of alcohol, cigarette smoking and other drugs to the unborn baby; and the dangers of passive smoking should be discussed. Maternal illnesses and medications should be reviewed.
   B. Information about the benefits of breast feeding or information about infant formula is provided. The use of car seats, safety of cribs, and issues regarding circumcision of boys should be discussed.

Prenatal Pediatric Visit Discussion Issues

Maternal History
   General health and nutrition
   Past and present obstetric history
   Maternal smoking, alcohol, or drug use
   Maternal medications
   Infectious diseases: Hepatitis, herpes, syphilis, Chlamydia rubella
   Maternal blood type and Rh blood groups
Family History
Newborn Issues
   Assessment of basic parenting skills
   Feeding plan: Breast feeding vs formula
   Car seats
   Circumcision of male infant

II. **Delivery**
   A. **Neonatal resuscitation**
      1. All equipment must be set up and checked before delivery. The infant who fails to breath spontaneously at birth should be placed under a radiant warmer, dried, positioned to open the airway, mouth and nares suctioned, and gentle stimulation provided.
      2. The mouth should be suctioned first to prevent aspiration. Prolonged or overly vigorous suctioning may lead to bradycardia and should be avoided unless moderate-to-thick meconium is present in the airway.
      3. The infant born with primary apnea is most likely to respond to the stimulation of drying and gentle tapping of the soles of the feet. The infant who fails to respond rapidly to these measures is experiencing secondary apnea and requires positive pressure bag ventilation with oxygen.
      4. Adequate ventilation is assessed by looking for chest wall excursions and listening for air exchange. The heart rate should be assessed while positive pressure ventilation is being applied. If the heart rate does not increase rapidly after ventilation, chest compressions must be started by an assistant. If the infant fails to respond to these measures, intubation and medications are necessary. Epinephrine can be administered via the endotracheal tube. Apgar scores are used to assess the status of the infant

at 1 and 5 min following delivery.

Apgar Scoring System			
Sign	**0**	**1**	**2**
Heart rate	Absent	Slow (<100 beats/min)	100 beats/min or more
Respirations	Absent	Weak cry; hypo-ventilation	Strong cry
Muscle tone	Limp	Some flexion	Active motion
Reflex irritability	No response	Grimace	Cough or sneeze
Color	Blue or pale	Body pink; extremities blue	Completely pink

III. **Early routine care of the newborn**
   A. **Vitamin K** is given to the infant by intramuscular injection to prevent hemorrhagic disease of the newborn.
   B. **Ocular prophylaxis** against gonorrheal and chlamydial infection is administered after birth with erythromycin ophthalmic ointment.
   C. **Umbilical cord blood syphilis serology** is completed if there is no documented record of a negative third-trimester maternal test. Umbilical cord care consists of local application of triple dye or bacitracin ointment.
   D. **Hepatitis B Prophylaxis.** If the mother is hepatitis B surface antigen-positive, or if she has active hepatitis B, the infant should be given an IM injection of hepatitis B immune globulin and a course of three injections of hepatitis B vaccine (before hospital discharge, and at 1 and 6 months of age).

IV. **Physical examination of the newborn**
   A. **General gestalt.** The examiner should assess whether the infant appears to be sick or well. An unusual cry may indicate sepsis, hypothyroidism, a congenital anomaly of the larynx, or a chromosomal abnormality.
   B. **Vital signs.** The normal temperature of the newborn is 36.5 to 37.0 degrees C. The normal respiratory rate ranges from 40 to 60 breaths per minute, and the normal heart rate can range from 94 to 175 beats per minute.
   C. **Assessment of the adequacy of fetal growth**
      1. **Gestational age assessment.** The gestational age of the newborn infant is assessed with the Ballard score of neuromuscular and physical maturity.
      2. **Premature infants**
         a. A preterm infant is defined as an infant of less than 37 weeks' gestation, and a postterm infant is defined as being of greater than 42 weeks' gestation.
         b. Preterm infants may develop respiratory distress syndrome, apnea, bradycardia, and retinopathy of prematurity. Respiratory distress syndrome is recognized by tachypnea, grunting, retractions, an elevated oxygen requirement, and a roentgenographic picture of poor inflation and a fine homogeneous ground-glass appearance.

D. Premature infants of less than 34-1/2 to 35 weeks' gestation are at increased risk for apnea and bradycardia. Apnea is defined as a respiratory pause of 20 sec or longer and frequently is accompanied by a drop in heart rate.

E. Measurements and growth charts

1. Height, weight, and head circumference should be measured. A low-birthweight infant is defined as any neonate with a birthweight <2,500 g. Height, weight, and head circumference should be plotted as a function of gestational age on an intrauterine growth chart.

2. Factors that may result in an infant who is small for gestational age include chromosomal and other dysmorphic syndromes, congenital infections, maternal hypertension, smoking, uterine anomalies, and multiple gestations.

3. The small-for-gestational age infant is at greater risk for cold stress, hypoglycemia, hypocalcemia, and polycythemia.

4. The differential diagnosis for the large-for-gestational age infant includes maternal diabetes and maternal obesity. The large-for-gestational age infant is at risk for shoulder dystocia, birth trauma, and hypoglycemia.

F. Examination of organ systems and regions

1. **Head, face, and neck**

   a. **The head circumference** is measured and plotted, and the scalp, fontanelles, and sutures are examined. Bruising and hematomas of the scalp should be noted. Cephalohematomas are subperiosteal and do not cross suture lines, whereas caputs are subcutaneous and do cross suture lines. An enlarged posterior fontanelle may be a sign of congenital hypothyroidism.

   b. **Facial features** that suggest a chromosomal anomaly include midfacial hypoplasia, small eyes, or low-set ears. Fetal alcohol syndrome is suggested by a small upper lip and a smooth philtrum.

   c. **The eyes** should be examined with an ophthalmoscope to document a red reflex. The absence of a clear red reflex is indicative of a retinoblastoma, cataract, or glaucoma.

   d. **The lips, mouth, and palate** are inspected and palpated for clefts. **Nares patency** can be documented by closing the mouth and occluding one nostril at a time while observing air flow through the opposite nostril.

2. **Thorax and cardiovascular systems**

   a. **Chest wall excursions** should be observed and the respiratory rate determined. The normal neonatal respiratory rate is 40 to 60 breaths per minute.

   b. **Auscultation of breath and heart sounds.** The normal heart rate during the first week of life may range from 94 to 175 beats per minute. The brachial and femoral pulses should be examined simultaneously to diagnose aortic coarctation.

3. **Abdomen and gastrointestinal system**

   a. **Visual inspection of the abdomen** should assess symmetry and distension.

   b. **Abdominal palpation** for masses, hepatosplenomegaly, or renal masses is completed, and the anus should be visually inspected.

4. **Genitourinary system.** The genitalia are examined for ambiguous genitalia, which requires immediate endocrinologic and urologic consultation.

5. **Musculoskeletal system**

   a. **Hip examination** may detect developmental dysplasia. Risk factors for hip dysplasia include a family history, foot deformities, congenital torticollis, Down syndrome, and breech presentation. The female to male ratio is 7:1. Ultrasonography is used to evaluate suspected hip dysplasia.

b. **Fracture of the clavicle** occurs in 0.2-3.5% of vaginal deliveries. Physical findings include local swelling and crepitations and an asymmetric Moro reflex. Treatment consists of making a sling by pinning the shirt sleeve of the involved side to the opposite side of the shirt.

6. **Neurologic system**

a. The degree of alertness, activity, and muscle tone should be noted. The head circumference is plotted on the growth chart.

b. The posterior midline area should be examined for evidence of neural tube defects. Pilonidal dimples with tufts of hair or no visible floor are evaluated with ultrasonography.

V. **Common neonatal problems**

A. **Hypoglycemia**

1. Hypoglycemia is common in premature infants, infants who are small for gestational age, infants of diabetic mothers, and infants who have experienced perinatal asphyxia.

2. Hypoglycemia is defined as a blood glucose of <40-45 mg/dL (<2.2-2.5 mmol/L). Hypoglycemic infants require early feedings or IV glucose.

B. **Anemia** during the newborn period may be caused by hemolytic and congenital anemias, fetal-to-maternal hemorrhage, placental abruption, and occult hemorrhage.

C. **Bilirubin metabolism**

1. Hyperbilirubinemia occurs frequently in the normal newborn because of increased production and decreased elimination of this breakdown product of heme.

2. Initial workup for neonatal hyperbilirubinemia includes measurements of total and direct bilirubin levels, hematocrit, Coombs test, and testing of urine for reducing substances to exclude galactosemia. High levels of bilirubin can cause an acute encephalopathy (ie, kernicterus).

D. **Sepsis** must be considered in any newborn who develops respiratory distress, temperature instability, hypoglycemia, lethargy, poor feeding, or jaundice. When sepsis is suspected, cultures of blood, urine, and spinal fluid are obtained. Antibiotic therapy must be initiated promptly.

E. **Gastrointestinal problems**

1. Ninety-six percent of full-term newborns pass a meconium stool before 24 hours of age. A delayed or absent passage of meconium may be caused by meconium plug syndrome, Hirschsprung disease, meconium ileus (cystic fibrosis), imperforate anus, or the small left colon syndrome (in infants of diabetic mothers).

2. Bilious vomiting in the newborn is always abnormal and usually is caused by an intestinal obstruction. Vomiting in the newborn also may be caused by inborn errors of metabolism and congenital adrenal hyperplasia.

F. **Urinary problems**. Ninety-nine percent of normal full-term infants will urinate by 24 hours. If urination has not occurred within 24 hours, renal ultrasonography should be done and an intravenous fluid challenge may be given.

References, see page 182.

Neonatal Jaundice

Jaundice is defined by a serum bilirubin concentration greater than 5 mg/dL. Clinical jaundice develops in 50% of newborns, and breast-feed infants have an increased incidence of jaundice. Differentiation between physiologic jaundice, which is seen in many infants during the first week of life, and pathologic jaundice is essential because pathologic jaundice is a sign of a more serious condition.

I. Pathophysiology
  A. Physiologic versus pathologic jaundice
     1. **Physiologic jaundice** is characterized by unconjugated hyperbilirubinemia that peaks by the third or fourth day of life in full-term newborns and then steadily declines by 1 week of age. Asian newborns tend to have higher peak bilirubin concentrations and more prolonged jaundice. Premature infants are more likely to develop jaundice than full-term babies.
     2. **Causes of physiologic jaundice**
        a. **Increased bilirubin load** due to the high red blood cell volume in newborns and shortened blood cell survival
        b. **Deficient hepatic uptake** and deficient conjugation of bilirubin
        c. **Increased enterohepatic bilirubin** reabsorption
        d. **Deficient excretion** of bilirubin.
     3. **Pathologic jaundice** usually appears within the first 24 hours after birth and is characterized by a rapidly rising serum bilirubin concentration (>5 mg/dL per day), prolonged jaundice (>7 to 10 days in a full-term infant), or an elevated direct bilirubin concentration (>2 mg/dL). Conjugated hyperbilirubinemia never has a physiologic cause and must always be investigated.
II. Clinical evaluation of jaundice in newborns
  A. **History** may reveal abdominal distention, delayed passage of meconium, lethargy, light colored stools, dark urine, low Apgar scores, poor feeding, weight loss, or vomiting.
  B. **Physical examination** should seek bruising, cephalhematoma, congenital anomalies, hepatosplenomegaly, pallor, petechiae, or small or large size for gestational age.
  C. **Maternal history** should assess history of chorioamnionitis, forceps delivery, vacuum extraction, diabetes, dystocia, or exposure to drugs. Failure to receive immune globulin in a previous pregnancy or abortion that involved risk of isoimmunization should be sought. Family history of jaundice, anemia, liver disease, splenectomy, Greek or Asian race, preeclampsia, or unexplained illness during pregnancy should be assessed.
III. Laboratory evaluation
  A. **Diagnostic tests** include blood group typing of both mother and infant, a direct Coombs' test, and measurement of serum bilirubin concentration.
  B. **Ill or premature infants**, or those with significant jaundice (serum bilirubin >15 mg/dL) require a complete blood cell count or hemoglobin, reticulocyte count, blood smear, and direct bilirubin level. In infants of Asian or Greek descent, glucose-6-phosphate dehydrogenase (G6PD) should be measured.
IV. Differential diagnosis of unconjugated hyperbilirubinemia
  A. Increased bilirubin production
     1. **Fetal-maternal blood group incompatibility** is one cause of increased bilirubin production. Rh sensitization occurs when an Rh-negative mother is exposed to Rh-positive blood cells. Subsequent Rh-positive fetuses may

develop hemolysis. Other minor blood group incompatibilities also can cause hemolysis and jaundice.

2. **ABO incompatibility** is the most common type of isoimmune hemolytic disease. It can occur when the mother's blood group is O and the baby's is A or B. This type of hemolysis is relatively mild.

3. **G6PD deficiency**, a sex-linked disease, is an important cause of hyperbilirubinemia and anemia in infants of Greek and Asian descent.

4. **Abnormalities of the red blood cell membrane**, such as spherocytosis and elliptocytosis, may cause hyperbilirubinemia. Alpha thalassemia may occur in the neonatal period.

5. **Hematoma, occult hemorrhage, or polycythemia** (fetomaternal or twin-to-twin transfusion, delayed cord clamping, intrauterine growth retardation, or maternal diabetes) may lead to hyperbilirubinemia.

B. **Decreased bilirubin excretion**

1. **Delay in intestinal transit time**, because of decreased motility or bowel obstruction, increases the enterohepatic circulation. Relief of the obstruction results in a decline in bilirubin concentration.

2. **Crigler-Najjar syndrome** is a rare, inherited, lifelong deficiency of bilirubin excretion. Type I is autosomal recessive. Patients present with extreme jaundice (bilirubin concentration ≥ 25 mg/dL) and have a very high risk of bilirubin encephalopathy. Type II is autosomal dominant, and it can effectively be treated with phenobarbital.

3. **Neonatal hypothyroidism** is another cause of prolonged indirect hyperbilirubinemia.

C. **Increased bilirubin production and decreased excretion**

1. Sepsis often causes increased breakdown of red blood cells and decreased hepatic excretion of bilirubin.

2. Certain drugs given to the newborn may also induce hemolysis or decrease bilirubin excretion.

D. **Breast feeding**

1. Feeding with breast milk is associated with neonatal hyperbilirubinemia.

2. In healthy newborns, the danger of an elevated bilirubin concentration is minimal, and switching to formula feeding is unnecessary.

V. **Consequences of unconjugated hyperbilirubinemia. Bilirubin encephalopathy (kernicterus)** is defined as the acute and often fatal syndrome characterized by opisthotonos, hypotonia, a high-pitched cry, and late neurologic sequelae of choreoathetosis, spasticity, upward-gaze paresis, and central hearing loss.

VI. **Treatment**

A. **Low-risk infants** with minimal jaundice are observed for an increase in the jaundice intensity or a spread to the baby's feet (jaundice advances from head-to-foot).

Management of Hyperbilirubinemia in the Healthy Term Newborn				
	Total serum bilirubin level, mg/dL			
Age (H)	Consider phototherapy	Phototherapy	Exchange transfusion if phototherapy fails	Exchange transfusion and photo-therapy
≤24	...	...	...	...
25-48	≥12	≥15	≥20	≥25
49-72	≥15	≥18	≥25	≥30
>72	≥17	≥20	≥25	≥30

B. **Phototherapy** with blue light causes photoconversion of bilirubin to a water-soluble product that is excreted in urine and stool. Bilirubin concentrations are measured once or twice a day during phototherapy, and treatment is discontinued when the bilirubin concentration drops below 12 mg/dL.
C. **Exchange transfusion therapy**. Exchange transfusion is used for emergent treatment of markedly elevated bilirubin and for correction of anemia caused by isoimmune hemolytic disease.

References, see page 182.

Respiratory Disorders of the Newborn

Respiratory distress is a common problem during the first few days of life. Respiratory distress may present with tachypnea, nasal flaring, sternal and intercostal retractions, cyanosis, and apnea.

I. **Transient tachypnea of the newborn**
   A. Transient tachypnea of the newborn (TTN) usually presents as early respiratory distress in term or preterm infants. It is caused by delayed reabsorption of fetal lung fluid.
   B. TTN is a very common, and it is often seen following cesarean section because, compared with those born vaginally, babies born by cesarean section have delayed reabsorption of fetal lung fluid.
   C. **Symptoms of TTN** include tachypnea, retractions, nasal flaring, grunting, and cyanosis.
   D. **Arterial blood gas** reveals respiratory acidosis and mild-to-moderate hypoxemia.
   E. **Chest x-ray** often reveals fluid in the interlobar fissures and perihilar streaking. Hyperaeration of the lungs and mild cardiomegaly may be seen; alveolar edema may appear as coarse, fluffy densities.
   F. Transient tachypnea of the newborn usually resolves within 12-24 hours. The chest radiograph appears normal in 2-3 days. The symptoms rarely last more

than 72 hours.

    G. **Treatment of TTN** consists of oxygen therapy. Infants will usually recover fully, without long-term pulmonary sequelae.

II. Respiratory distress syndrome

A. RDS is a lung disease caused by pulmonary surfactant deficiency. It occurs almost always in preterm infants who are born before the lungs are able to produce adequate amounts of surfactant.

B. Respiratory distress usually begins at, or soon after, delivery and tends to worsen over time. Infants will have tachypnea, nasal flaring, intercostal and sternal retractions, and expiratory grunting. Tiny preterm infants who lack pulmonary surfactant may fail to initiate ventilation in the delivery room.

C. **Chest radiography** shows diffuse atelectasis, which appears as reduced lung volume, with homogeneous haziness or the "ground glass" appearance of lung fields, and air bronchograms.

D. RDS is diagnosed when a premature infant has respiratory distress and a characteristic chest radiograph. The differential diagnosis includes pneumonia, often caused by group B streptococci.

E. **Ventilatory management**

    1. Continuous positive airway pressure (CPAP) improves oxygenation and survival (5-7 cm H_2O pressure).

    2. For infants exhibiting respiratory acidosis, hypoxemia or apnea, intermittent positive pressure ventilation will be required in addition to positive end-expiratory pressure (PEEP).

    3. An umbilical or radial arterial line is used to monitor blood gas levels and blood pressure in sicker infants.

F. **Surfactant replacement therapy**

    1. Surfactant therapy reduces mortality by 30-50% and pneumothorax by 50%.

    2. Surfactant replacement therapy should be initiated as soon as respiratory distress has been clinically diagnosed. As long as the infant requires significant ventilatory support, including more than 30% oxygen, Survanta (every 6 hours for 4 doses) or Exosurf (every 12 hours for 2 doses) should be given.

G. **General supportive care**

    1. Sepsis and pneumonia are part of the differential diagnosis of RDS. Presumptive treatment with ampicillin plus gentamicin or cefotaxime usually is given until blood and CSF cultures are negative.

    2. Restricting intravenous fluid in infants who have RDS lowers the risk for development of bronchopulmonary dysplasia. Systemic blood pressure should be maintained in the normal range with dopamine (3-20 mg/kg/min IV) or dobutamine (2.5-15.0 mg/kg/min IV based on response).

III. Bronchopulmonary dysplasia

A. Bronchopulmonary dysplasia (BPD) is a chronic lung disease characterized by hypoxia, hypercarbia, and oxygen dependence that persists beyond 1 month of age. The chest radiograph shows hyperexpansion and focal hyperlucency, alternating with strands of opacification.

B. BPD is extremely common among infants who have severe RDS treated with mechanical ventilation. The incidence of BPD is inversely proportional to birthweight. Virtually all babies who develop BPD have had mechanical ventilation, suggesting an important role for barotrauma and oxygen toxicity.

C. RDS is the most common pulmonary disease causing BPD. Other neonatal diseases requiring oxygen and mechanical ventilation may also cause BPD, including immature lungs, meconium aspiration syndrome, congenital heart disease, neonatal pneumonia, and aspiration pneumonia.

D. Signs of BPD include tachypnea and retractions, after extubation. Blood gas measurements show respiratory acidosis with elevated $PaVCO_2$; increased HCO_3 indicates metabolic compensation. Higher inspired oxygen concentration is required to maintain normal oxygenation.

E. Management of BPD consists of minimizing barotrauma. Adjustments in peak pressure should deliver adequate, but not excessive, tidal volume; acceptable minute ventilation can be maintained by monitoring the $PaCO_2$. A moderate degree of respiratory acidosis should be allowed in order to decrease the amount of ventilatory assistance needed, thus reducing the barotrauma. Supplemental oxygen therapy should maintain the PaO_2 in the 60-80 mm Hg range.

F. **Nutrition** is crucial in promoting repair and growth of lung tissue. Infants who have BPD may not tolerate even normal fluid intakes. These infants may need up to 150 kcal/kg/day for optimal growth.

G. **Antibiotics.** Intubated infants who have BPD are susceptible to pneumonia. Close observation for pneumonia and prompt treatment with antibiotics, when pneumonia is suspected, are recommended.

H. **Chest physiotherapy**, with chest percussion, postural drainage and suctioning should be performed as needed.

I. **Diuretic therapy.** Furosemide (1 mg/kg q 24 h IV or PO) may be used. Milder diuretics such as chlorothiazide (10-20 mg/kg per dose q12h PO) and spironolactone (1-2 mg/kg per dose q12h PO) may help reduce airway resistance and improve pulmonary compliance.

J. **Bronchodilators**
   1. Aminophylline (5-7 mg/kg loading dose, followed by 2 mg/kg q6-12h IV) decreases airway resistance and increases lung compliance.
   2. Inhaled albuterol, 0.15 mg/kg q 8 h, has been shown to benefit pulmonary function.

K. **Corticosteroid Therapy.** Dexamethasone (0.25 mg/kg q12h PO or IV for 3 days, followed by a tapering course over 2-6 weeks) has been shown to improve pulmonary function rapidly and allow earlier extubation.

L. **Home oxygen therapy** should be considered for infants who are receiving supplemental oxygen therapy.

References, see page 182.

Neonatal Resuscitation

Neonatal resuscitation skills are important because of the potential for serious disability or death in high-risk infants and in a few unpredicted full-term, low-risk deliveries.

I. **Preparation**
   A. **Advanced preparation** requires acquisition and maintenance of proper equipment and supplies.
   B. **Immediate preparation**
      1. Suction, oxygen, proper-sized face mask and the resuscitation bag should be checked.
      2. Appropriately sized ET tubes, cut to 13 cm, should be laid out.
      3. Medications should be prepared and an umbilical catheter and tray should be prepared.

Neonatal Resuscitation Equipment and Supplies

Suction Equipment

Bulb syringe
Suction catheters, 5 (or 6), 8, 10 Fr
Meconium aspirator

Mechanical Suction
8 Fr feeding tube and 20 cc syringe

Bag-and-Mask Equipment

Oral airways, newborn and premature sizes
Infant resuscitation bag with a pressure-release valve/pressure gauge to give 90-100% O_2

Oxygen with flow meter and tubing
Cushion rim face masks in newborn and premature sizes

Intubation Equipment

Laryngoscope with straight blades, No. O (preterm) and No.1(term newborn).
Extra bulbs and batteries for laryngoscope
Endotracheal tubes, size 2.5, 3.0, 3.5, 4.0 mm

Stylet
Scissors
Gloves

Medications

Epinephrine 1:10,000, 3 cc or 10 cc ampules
Naloxone 0.4 mg/mL,1 mL ampules
Dextrose 10% in water, 250 cc
Sterile water, 30 cc

Volume expanders-one or more of these:
    Albumin 5% solution
    Normal Saline
    Ringer's Lactate solution

Miscellaneous

Radiant warmer and towels or blankets
Stethoscope
Adhesive tape, ½ or 3/4 inch width
Syringes, 1 cc, 3 cc, 5 cc, 10 cc, 20 cc, 50 cc
Umbilical artery catheterization tray
Cardiotachometer and ECG oscilloscope

Alcohol sponges
3-way stopcocks
3 Fr feeding tube
Umbilical tape
Needles, 25, 21, 18 gauge
Umbilical catheters, 3 ½ and 5 Fr

II. **Neonatal resuscitation procedures**
    A. **During delivery**, infant evaluation includes assessment of muscle tone, color, and respiratory effort.
    B. **After delivery**, the infant should be placed on a preheated radiant warmer. The infant should be quickly dried with warm towels. The infant should be placed supine with its neck in a neutral position. A towel neck roll under the shoulders may help prevent neck flexion and airway occlusion.
    C. The **upper airway is cleared** by suctioning; the mouth first, and then the nose, using a bulb syringe. Suctioning should be limited to 5 seconds at a time.
    D. If breathing is effective and pulse is ≥100 beats/min, positive pressure ventilation (PPV) is not needed. If cyanosis is present, oxygen should be administered.
    E. **Free-flowing oxygen** may be given at a rate of 5 L/min by holding the tubing ½ inch in front of the infant's nose or an oxygen mask may be used. When the infant's color is pink, the oxygen is gradually discontinued.
    F. **Positive pressure ventilation** should be initiated if the infant is not breathing effectively after the initial steps. Tactile stimulation should be administered by gently slapping the soles of the feet or rubbing the back. If the infant is apneic or gasping, begin PPV with 100% O_2. If the heart rate is <100 beats/min, give PPV immediately by bag-mask.
       1. **Bag-Mask ventilation.** The first ventilations should be given at a rate of 40-60/min. Visible chest wall movement indicates adequate ventilation.
       2. **Endotracheal intubation** is initiated if the infant is nonresponsive to bag-mask PPV.

Endotracheal Tube Size and Depth of Insertion From Upper Lip

Weight	Gestational Age	Size	Depth
<1000 g	<28 weeks	2.5 mm	7 cm
1000-2000 g	28-34 weeks	3.0 mm	8 cm
2000-3000 g	34-38 weeks	3.5 mm	9 cm
3000 g or more	39-≥40 weeks	4.0 mm	10 cm

    G. **Evaluation of heart rate**
       1. If the heart rate is ≥100 beats/min, PPV can be gradually discontinued after the infant is breathing effectively.
       2. **Chest compressions** should be started if the heart rate is <80 beats/min after 15-30 seconds of adequate ventilation.
          a. Chest compressions are alternated with ventilations at a ratio of 3:1. The combined rate should be 120/min (ie, 80 compressions and 30 ventilations). After 30 seconds, evaluate the response. If the pulse is ≥80 beats/min, chest compressions can be stopped and PPV continued until the heart rate is 100 beats/min and effective breathing is maintained.
       3. **Epinephrine** should be given if the heart rate remains below 80/minute after 30 seconds of PPV and chest compressions.

Neonatal Resuscitation Medications				
Medication	Concentration	Preparation	Dosage	Rate/Precautions
Epinephrine	1:10,000	1 mL	0.1-0.3 mL/kg IV or ET. May repeat in 3-5 min if HR is <80/min	Give rapidly. May dilute 1:1 with normal saline if given via ET
Volume expanders	Whole blood Albumin 5% Normal saline Ringer lactate	40 mL	10 mL/kg IV	Give over 5-10 min by syringe or IV drip
Naloxone	0.4 mg/mL	1 mL	0.1 mg/kg (0.25 mL/kg) IV, ET, IM, SQ	Give rapidly
Naloxone	1.0 mg/mL	1 mL	1 mg/kg (0.1 mL/kg) IV, ET, IM, SQ	IV, ET preferred. IM, SQ acceptable
Sodium bicarbonate	0.5 mEq/mL (4.2% solution) diluted with sterile water to make 0.5 mEq/mL	20 mL or two 10-mL prefilled syringes	2 mEq/kg IV	Give slowly, over at least 2 min.

4. **Other medications**
   a. **Volume expanders.** Volume expansion is indicated for patients who have known or suspected blood loss and poor response to other resuscitative measures. Albumin 5%, normal saline, or Ringer's lactate can be given in boluses of 10 mL/kg over 5 to 10 minutes.
   b. **Sodium bicarbonate** is recommended during prolonged resuscitation for infants refractory to other measures.
   c. **Naloxone hydrochloride** is given to infants with prolonged respiratory depression following narcotic anesthesia given to the mother within 4 hrs before delivery. Naloxone is contraindicated in infants of mothers who are addicted to narcotics.
5. **Umbilical vessel catheterization** is recommended when vascular access is required. The large, centrally located, thin-walled and flat vein is used, and a 3.5 or 5.0 Fr radiopaque catheter is inserted into the vein until a free flow of blood can be aspirated.

References, see page 182.

General Pediatrics

Diabetes Mellitus

Diabetes mellitus consists of hyperglycemia caused by insulin deficiency, impairment of insulin action, or both. Five percent of the population is affected by diabetes, 10% of whom have type 1 diabetes.

I.   **Classification of diabetes mellitus**
   A. Diabetes mellitus is classified into two types: type 1 and type 2.
   B. **Type 1 diabetes**
       1. Type 1 diabetes is caused by absolute insulin deficiency. Most cases among children and adolescents (95%) result from autoimmune destruction of the beta cells of the pancreas.
       2. The peak age at diagnosis is 12 years, and 75-80% of individuals develop type 1 diabetes before age 30.
   C. **Type 2 diabetes**
       1. Type 2 diabetes is caused by insulin resistance and relative insulin deficiency. Most type 2 diabetics do not require insulin injections. Most patients who have type 2 diabetes are obese.

II. **Pathogenesis of type 1 diabetes**
   A. Type 1 diabetes develops in individuals who are genetically susceptible, have certain environmental exposures, and have immune-mediated destruction of the beta cells.
   B. Although 80-85% of patients who have type 1 diabetes have no other affected family member, the relative risk increases to 1 in 20 (from 1 in 300) for first-degree relatives.

III. **Clinical presentation of type 1 diabetes**
   A. **Classic signs and symptoms of diabetes** include polyuria, polydipsia, and polyphagia. Extremely high glucose levels cause a severe diuresis that results in fluid, electrolyte, and calorie loss.

Criteria for Diagnosis of Diabetes

Fasting plasma glucose 126 mg/dL or higher
or
Random plasma glucose 200 mg/dL or higher with symptoms of diabetes (fatigue, weight loss, polyuria, polyphagia, polydipsia)
or
Abnormal two-hour 75-g oral glucose tolerance test result, with glucose 200 mg/dL or higher at two hours
Any abnormal test result must be repeated on a subsequent occasion to establish the diagnosis

---

IV. **Management of diabetic ketoacidosis**
   A. DKA can be seen at the time of diagnosis of type 1 diabetes or in the patient who has established disease if diabetes management is inadequate.
   B. DKA is caused by insulin deficiency, which leads to hyperglycemia and ketogenesis.
   C. **Symptoms** include polyuria, polydipsia, hyperpnea with shortness of breath,

vomiting, and abdominal pain. Hyperosmolar dehydration and acid/base and electrolyte disturbances occur. In the advanced stages of DKA, the level of consciousness alters and can lead to coma.

D. **Rehydration**
1. **Immediate evaluation** should assess the degree of dehydration by determining capillary refill, skin temperature, and postural heart rate and blood pressure.
2. Initial fluid resuscitation consists of a 10-mL/kg bolus of 0.9% saline over 30-60 minutes, repeated if hypovolemic shock persists. Patients then should begin to receive maintenance fluid requirements (1,500 mL/m² per 24 h) added to the calculated fluid deficit (>2 y: 30 mL/kg for mild deficit, 60 mL/kg for moderate deficit, 90 mL/kg for severe deficit; <2 y: 50 mL/kg for mild deficit, 100 mL/kg for moderate deficit, 150 mL/kg for severe deficit). The sodium concentration of the fluid should provide 50% of the sodium deficit in the first 12 hours and the remainder in the next 36 hours (75 to 125 mEq/L sodium chloride).
3. Excessive fluid administration and inadequate sodium replacement in the first 24 hours of therapy can lead to a decrease in serum osmolality and cerebral edema.

Laboratory Monitoring During DKA	
Blood glucose:	At presentation, then hourly by fingerstick with glucose meter
Serum sodium and potassium:	At presentation, then at 4- to 6-h intervals
Acid/base status:	At presentation, then at 2- to 4-h intervals. Venous pH and serum carbon dioxide
Serum urea nitrogen, complete blood count, acetone and appropriate cultures can be obtained at presentation.	

E. **Potassium replacement**
1. DKA is associated with total body potassium depletion. This deficit should be replaced by infusing potassium chloride at a rate of 3 mEq/kg per 24 hours after completion of the normal saline fluid resuscitation.
2. If the patient requires more than 4 mEq/kg of a potassium infusion, 50% can be administered as potassium phosphate to help prevent hyperchloremic acidosis and hypophosphatemia.
F. **Lowering the glucose level**
1. Regular insulin should be initiated as an intravenous infusion of 0.1 U/kg per hour. The goal of therapy is to lower the glucose level by 50 to 100 mg/dL per hour.
2. Once the glucose level is in the range of 250 to 350 mg/dL, 5% glucose should be initiated; when the glucose level is between 180 to 240 mg/dL, the infusate can be changed to 10% glucose.
G. **Correcting acidosis.** Alkali therapy is usually not necessary to correct the acidosis associated with DKA. If acidosis is severe, with a pH less than 7.1, sodium bicarbonate can be infused slowly at a rate of 1 to 3 mEq/kg per 12

hours and discontinued when the pH exceeds 7.2.

H. Cerebral edema

1. Cerebral edema is a potentially life-threatening complication in 2-3% of cases of DKA. The typical presentation is acute neurologic deterioration 6 to 12 hours after the initiation of treatment, although some patients have antecedent headache, lethargy, incontinence, seizures, pupillary changes, and signs of intracranial hypertension.

2. Cerebral edema is treated with mannitol (0.25 to 1.0 g/kg IV), which should be administered rapidly when neurologic symptoms develop.

V. Long-term diabetes management

A. Intensive management of diabetes results in a significant reduction in the development of diabetic complications: a 76% reduction in retinopathy, a 39% reduction in microalbuminuria, and a 60% reduction in neuropathy.

Target Blood Glucose Range (Preprandial)	
Age	**Glucose Levels (mg/dL)**
Infants, toddlers	120-220
Preschool children	100-200
School-age children	70-150

B. Insulin regimens

1. The preferred insulin preparation is human insulin. For preschool- and school-age children, two injections are usually all that is required to achieve targeted glycemia. Insulin is distributed as short-acting (regular insulin) and intermediate-acting (NPH) insulin before breakfast, and a small dose of regular and NPH insulin at dinner.

2. If indicated to improve morning blood glucose levels, the evening dosage can be split so that the short-acting insulin is administered before dinner and the intermediate-acting is administered before bedtime.

Total Daily Insulin Dosage		
<5 Years (U/kg)	**5-11 Years (U/kg)**	**12-18 Years (U/kg)**
0.6-0.8	0.75-0.9	0.8-1.5
Newly diagnosed patients and those who are in the remission phase may require less insulin. If the required dosage exceeds these guidelines, consider cryptic illness, causes of insulin resistance, or non-adherence.		

Meal Plans	
Calorie Content
2000 kcal/m^2 or 1000 kcal + 100 kcal/year of age	
Distribution	
25% Breakfast	
25% Lunch	
30% Dinner	
20% Snacks	
Food Type	
50% carbohydrate	
25% to 30% fat	
20% to 25% protein	

C. **Insulin analogs** have a more rapid onset of action than regular insulin. Lispro insulin has an onset of action of 10 minutes and a duration of action of 2 hours. The ability to administer lispro 10 minutes prior to eating improves lifestyle. In very young children, it may be given after the meal when the exact quantity of food ingested can be determined.

D. **Blood glucose monitoring.** Children and adolescents should test their blood glucose levels at least four times a day, before meals and at bedtime. Additional testing should be performed intermittently, particularly in the middle of the night and at times of unusual behavior in very young children. Quarterly measurement of hemoglobin A1c (HbA1c) assesses glycemic control and reflects the average blood glucose over the last 120 days.

Assessment of HbA1c Values	
HbA1c Values	**Level of Glycemic Control**
HbA1c >10%	Poor or minimal
HbA1c 8.0-10.0%	Average
<8.0%	Excellent or intensive

E. **Urinary microalbumin excretion** should be assessed with an albumin-to-creatinine ratio yearly, starting five years after diabetes has been diagnosed. If albumin is high--exceeding 30 mg/g on at least two occasions--the adequacy of glycemic control should be reevaluated.

F. **Thyroid function tests** should be obtained at diagnosis and when symptoms develop. There is an increased risk of autoimmune thyroiditis, and 6% of diabetic children also have hypothyroidism.

G. Five years after diagnosis, annual dilated ophthalmologic examination by an ophthalmologist should be initiated.

References, see page 182.

Menstrual Disorders

The median age of menarche is 12.8 years, and the normal menstrual cycle is 21 to 35 days in length. Bleeding normally lasts for 3 to 7 days and consists of 30 to 40 mL of blood. Cycles are abnormal if they are longer than 8 to 10 days or if more than 80 mL of blood loss occurs. Soaking more than 25 pads or 30 tampons during a menstrual period is abnormal.

I. Pathophysiology
   A. **Regular ovulatory menstrual cycles** often do not develop until 1 to 1.5 years after menarche, and 55-82% of cycles are anovulatory for the first 2 years after menarche. Anovulatory cycles typically cause heavier and longer bleeding.
   B. **Adolescents** frequently experience irregular menstrual bleeding patterns, which can include several consecutive months of amenorrhea.
   C. **The normal menstrual cycle**
      1. **During the follicular phase**, release of gonadotropin-releasing hormone (GnRH) from the hypothalamus stimulates the pituitary to secrete luteinizing hormone (LH) and follicle-stimulating hormone (FSH), which then stimulate ovarian estrogen secretion, which induces endometrial proliferation.
      2. **Ovulation** occurs 12 hours after the midcycle surge in LH.
      3. **The luteal phase** follows ovulation, and the corpus luteum secretes progesterone and estrogen. Progesterone inhibits endometrial proliferation and induces glandular changes. Without fertilization, progesterone and estradiol levels decrease, and sloughing of the endometrium occurs 14 days after ovulation.

II. Amenorrhea
   A. **Primary amenorrhea** is defined as the absence of menarche by age 16. Puberty is considered delayed and warrants evaluation if breast development (the initial sign of puberty in girls) does not begin by the age of 13. The mean time between the onset of breast development and menarche is 2 years. Absence of menses within 2 to 2.5 years of the onset of puberty should be evaluated.
   B. **Secondary amenorrhea** is defined as the absence of 3 consecutive menstrual cycles or 6 months of amenorrhea in patients who have already established regular menstrual periods.

Differential Diagnosis of Amenorrhea	
Pregnancy	**Outflow Tract-related Disorders**
Hormonal Contraception	Imperforate hymen
Hypothalamic-related Disorders	Transverse vaginal septum
Chronic or systemic illness	Agenesis of the vagina, cervix, uterus
Stress	Uterine synechiae
Athletics	**Androgen Excess**
Eating disorders	Polycystic ovarian syndrome
Obesity	Adrenal tumor
Drugs	Adrenal hyperplasia (classic and
Tumor	nonclassic)
Pituitary-related Disorders	Ovarian tumor
Hypopituitarism	**Other Endocrine Disorders**
Tumor	Thyroid disease
Infiltration	Cushing syndrome
Infarction	
Ovarian-related Disorders	
Dysgenesis	
Agenesis	
Ovarian failure	
Resistant ovary	

C. **Amenorrhea with pubertal delay**
   1. **Hypergonadotropic hypogonadism** is caused by ovarian failure associated with elevated gonadotropin levels. An elevated FSH will establish this diagnosis.
      a. **Turner syndrome (XO)** may cause ovarian failure and a lack of pubertal development. Females with Turner syndrome have streak gonads, absence of one of the X chromosomes, and inadequate levels of estradiol. They do not initiate puberty or uterine development. This syndrome is characterized by short stature, webbed neck, widely spaced nipples, shield chest, high arched palate, congenital heart disease, renal anomalies, and autoimmune disorders (thyroiditis, Addison disease). It may not be diagnosed until adolescence, when pubertal delay and amenorrhea occur together.
      b. **Ovarian failure** resulting from autoimmune disorders or exposure to radiation or chemotherapy may also cause amenorrhea with pubertal delay associated with hypergonadotropic hypogonadism.
   2. **Hypogonadotropic hypogonadism** is caused by hypothalamic dysfunction or pituitary failure. Low or normal levels of LH and FSH will be present, and decreased estradiol levels may be present.
      a. **Abnormalities of the pituitary and hypothalamus**, and other endocrinopathies (thyroid disease and Cushing syndrome) may present with pubertal delay and low gonadotropin levels.
         (1) Amenorrhea may be caused by problems at the level of the pituitary gland, such as congenital hypopituitarism, tumor (pituitary adenoma), or infiltration (hemochromatosis).
         (2) **Prolactin-secreting pituitary adenoma (prolactinoma)** is the most common pituitary tumor. Prolactinomas present with galactorrhea, headache, visual fields cuts, and amenorrhea. Elevated prolactin levels are characteristic.
         (3) **Craniopharyngioma** is another tumor of the sella turcica that affects hypothalamic-pituitary function, presenting with pubertal

delay and amenorrhea.

(4) Other disorders associated with galactorrhea and amenorrhea include hypothyroidism, breast stimulation, stress associated with trauma or surgery, phenothiazines, and opiates).

b. **Hypothalamic suppression** is most commonly caused by stress, competitive athletics, and inadequate nutrition (anorexia nervosa).

c. Hypothalamic abnormalities associated with pubertal delay include Laurence-Moon-Biedl, Prader-Willi, and Kallmann syndromes. Laurence-Moon-Biedl and Prader-Willi present with obesity. Kallmann syndrome is associated with anosmia.

D. **Amenorrhea with normal pubertal development**

1. **Pregnancy** should be excluded when amenorrhea occurs in a pubertally mature female.

2. **Contraceptive-related amenorrhea** occurs with depot medroxyprogesterone (Depo-Provera) and levonorgestrel implants (Norplant); it does not require intervention; however, a pregnancy test should be completed.

3. **Uterine synechiae (Asherman syndrome)** should be suspected in amenorrheic females with a history of abortion, dilation and curettage, or endometritis.

4. **Sheehan syndrome (pituitary infarction)** is suggested by a history of intrapartum bleeding and hypotension.

5. **Other disorders associated with amenorrhea and normal pubertal development.** Ovarian failure, acquired abnormalities of the pituitary gland (prolactinoma), thyroid disease, and stress, athletics, and eating disorders may cause amenorrhea after normal pubertal development. Polycystic ovarian disease, which is usually associated with irregular bleeding, can also present with amenorrhea.

E. **Genital tract abnormalities**

1. **Imperforate hymen** will appear as a membrane covering the vaginal opening. A history of cyclic abdominal pain is common, and a midline abdominal mass may be palpable.

2. **Transverse vaginal septum** may cause obstruction. It is diagnosed by speculum examination.

3. **Agenesis of the vagina** appears as a blind-ended pouch. Normal pubertal development of breast and pubic hair occurs, but menarche does not occur.

4. **Androgen insensitivity (testicular feminization syndrome)** is another common cause of vaginal agenesis.

a. Breast development and a growth spurt occur, but little if any pubic or axillary hair is present. These women have an XY chromosomal pattern with intra-abdominal or inguinal testes that produce testosterone, but an X-linked inherited defect of the androgen receptor prevents response to testosterone.

b. Female-appearing external genitalia are present, but the uterus and vagina are absent. During puberty, breast development occurs because of conversion of androgens to estrogens.

c. The testes are at increased risk for developing tumors and must be removed. Hormone replacement therapy is provided to initiate puberty.

F. **Polycystic ovary syndrome (hyperandrogenic anovulation)**

1. PCO is the most common cause of persistent irregular menses. Only 70% of patients have polycystic ovaries on ultrasound. The most common symptom is irregular periods beginning with menarche; however, intervals of amenorrhea may also occur. Signs include hirsutism, acne,

clitoromegaly, and obesity (50%). Insulin resistance, glucose intolerance, and lipid abnormalities are common.

2. Increased facial hair and midline hair over the sternum and lower abdomen are often present. If hirsutism is severe, an ovarian and adrenal tumor or adrenal enzyme deficiency should be excluded.

3. PCO is probably an autosomal recessive disorder that affects ovarian steroidogenesis. Ovulation occasionally can occur spontaneously; therefore, amenorrhea secondary to pregnancy always must be considered.

G. **Clinical evaluation of amenorrhea**

1. **Chronic or systemic illness**, eating disorders, and drug use, including hormonal contraception, should be excluded. Tanner staging, pelvic examination, and possibly pelvic ultrasonography should be completed.

2. **Absence of the uterus**, vagina, or both requires a chromosomal analysis, which can determine if the karyotype is XX or XY, and it can help differentiate between müllerian agenesis and androgen insensitivity.

3. If the anatomy is normal, LH, FSH, and estradiol are indicated in order to distinguish ovarian failure from hypothalamic dysfunction. High FSH and LH levels and a low estradiol level are indicators of gonadal dysgenesis (Turner syndrome) or autoimmune oophoritis. Normal or low LH, FSH, and estradiol levels indicate hypothalamic suppression, central nervous system tumor, or an endocrinopathy (eg, hypothyroidism).

4. **Pregnancy** must always be excluded if the individual is mature pubertally.

5. **Free-T4, TSH, and prolactin** levels are checked to exclude hypothyroidism and hyperprolactinemia. If the prolactin level is elevated, an MRI is necessary to exclude prolactinoma.

6. **Hirsutism and acne** are indicative of androgen excess and PCO. Total testosterone and dehydroepiandrosterone sulfate (DHEAS) levels are necessary to exclude ovarian and adrenal tumors. A testosterone level >200 ng/dL and DHEAS >700 µg/dL require further investigation to exclude a tumor.

7. **A morning 17-hydroxyprogesterone level** will screen for nonclassic adrenal hyperplasia. A 17-hydroxyprogesterone >2 ng/mL is followed by an ACTH stimulation test to diagnose 21-hydroxylase deficiency.

8. An elevated LH-to-FSH ratio is common with PCO; an ultrasonographic examination may detect polycystic ovaries.

H. **Treatment of amenorrhea**

1. **Anovulation** and the resulting lack of progesterone increases the risk of endometrial hyperplasia and endometrial cancer. Oral medroxyprogesterone or an oral contraceptive (OCs) should be prescribed to eliminate this risk. Oral progestins can be given cyclically for 12 days every month or every third month.

2. **PCO** is treated with OCs to regulate menses and to decrease androgen levels. Electrolysis and spironolactone (50 mg tid) can decrease hirsutism.

3. **Hypoestrogenic and anovulatory patients** with hypothalamic suppression caused by anorexia, stress, or strenuous athletics should modify their behavior and be prescribed calcium and hormonal replacement therapy (OCs) to reduce the risks of osteoporosis.

4. **Turner syndrome or ovarian failure** requires estrogen and progesterone at a dosage sufficient to induce pubertal development, after which time they can be switched to an OC.

III. **Abnormal vaginal bleeding**

    A. Abnormal vaginal bleeding is characterized by excessive uterine bleeding or a prolonged number of days of bleeding. The most common cause of abnormal vaginal bleeding in adolescence is anovulation. Abnormal bleeding is common during the first 1 to 2 years after menarche because anovulatory cycles are frequent.

    B. **Differential diagnosis of abnormal vaginal bleeding**

        1. **Pregnancy**, pregnancy-related complications, sexually transmitted diseases, pelvic inflammatory disease, and retained tampons should be excluded.

        2. **Vaginal tumors**, uterine or cervical carcinoma, and uterine myomas are rare in adolescents.

        3. **Blood dyscrasias or coagulation defects** may occasionally be the initial presentation of abnormal vaginal bleeding.

        4. **Hormonal contraceptives** are a common cause of breakthrough bleeding.

    C. **Clinical evaluation of irregular vaginal bleeding**

        1. Age of menarche, menstrual pattern, amount of bleeding, symptoms of hypovolemia, history of sexual activity, genital trauma, and symptoms of endocrine abnormalities or systemic illness should be evaluated.

        2. Postural vital signs may suggest hypovolemia. A pelvic examination should assess pelvic anatomy and exclude trauma, infection, foreign body, or a pregnancy-related complication. Pelvic ultrasonography can be used to further assess pelvic anatomy.

Differential Diagnosis of Abnormal Vaginal Bleeding

Pregnancy-related. Ectopic pregnancy, abortion

Hormonal contraception. Oral contraceptives, depo-medroxyprogesterone

Hypothalamic-related. Chronic or systemic illness, stress, athletics, eating disorder, obesity, drugs

Pituitary-related. Prolactinoma, craniopharyngioma

Outflow tract-related. Trauma, foreign body, vaginal tumor, cervical carcinoma, polyp, uterine myoma, uterine carcinoma, intrauterine device

Androgen excess. Polycystic ovarian syndrome, adrenal tumor, ovarian tumor, adrenal hyperplasia

Other endocrine causes. Thyroid disease, adrenal disease

Hematologic causes. Thrombocytopenia, clotting abnormalities, abnormalities of platelet function, anticoagulant medications

Infectious causes. Pelvic inflammatory disease, cervicitis

---

        3. **Laboratory evaluation**

            a. **A pregnancy test and complete blood count** should be completed.

            b. **A history of a very heavy period with menarche** or repeated prolonged or heavy menses warrants a prothrombin time and partial thromboplastin time to screen for bleeding abnormalities; a bleeding time and von Willebrand screening panel will identify more specific coagulation disorders.

            c. **Signs of androgen excess** indicate a need to exclude PCO.

            d. **Chronic irregular vaginal bleeding** mandates that prolactinoma and endocrine abnormalities (thyroid disease) be excluded.

    D. Treatment of irregular vaginal bleeding

        1. **Mild bleeding or shortened cycles** associated with a normal physical examination and normal vital signs requires only reassurance.

        2. **Mild anemia** associated with stable vital signs is treated with a 35 to 50 mcg monophasic combination OC as follows: One pill QID x 4 days. One pill TID x 3 days. One pill BID x 7 days. One pill QD x 7-14 days. Stop all pills for 7 days and then begin cycling on a low dose OCP QD.

        3. The patient should be continued on low-dose OCs for 3 to 4 months before allowing resumption of normal cycles. Iron therapy should be included.

        4. **If the hematocrit is <7-8 mg/dL or if vital signs are unstable,** hospitalization is recommended. Intravenous conjugated estrogens (Premarin), 25 mg IV every 4-6 hours for 24 hours, will stop the bleeding quickly. Conjugated estrogen therapy is followed immediately by OCs and iron therapy. Blood transfusion is warranted only if the patient is severely symptomatic. Dilatation and curettage is used as a last resort; however, it is rarely necessary.

        5. **Antiprostaglandin medications (NSAIDs)** decrease menstrual blood loss significantly by promoting platelet aggregation and vasoconstriction. They do not cause the hormonal side effects of OCs, and they can be used alone in mild cases of abnormal vaginal bleeding.

IV. Dysmenorrhea

    A. Fifty percent of adolescents experience dysmenorrhea

    B. Primary dysmenorrhea consists of crampy lower abdominal and pelvic pain during menses that is not associated with pelvic pathology. It is the most common form of dysmenorrhea, usually beginning 6 months to 1 year after menarche.

    C. Secondary dysmenorrhea is defined as painful menses associated with pelvic pathology (bicornate uterus, endometriosis, PID, uterine fibroids and polyps, cervical stenosis, ovarian neoplasms). If dysmenorrhea is severe, obstructing lesions of the genital tract should be excluded. Endometriosis is the most common cause (50%) of chronic pelvic pain in adolescents.

    D. Evaluation of dysmenorrhea

        1. **Gynecologic history** should determine the relationship of the pain to the menstrual cycle, severity, and sexual activity.

        2. **If the pain is mild,** easily relieved by NSAIDs, and the physical examination (including the hymen) are normal, a speculum examination is not necessary.

        3. **Severe pain** requires a pelvic examination to exclude genital tract obstruction, adnexal and/or uterosacral pain (endometriosis), PID, or a mass. Ultrasonography is useful for evaluating pelvic abnormalities or obstruction.

    E. Treatment of dysmenorrhea

        1. **Initial treatment** consists of a prostaglandin synthesis inhibitor, initiated with the onset of bleeding and continued for as long as pain lasts. Gastric irritation can be reduced by taking the drug with food.

            a. **Mefenamic acid (Ponstel)** 500 mg loading dose, then 250 mg q6h.

            b. **Ibuprofen (Advil)** 400-600 mg q4-6h.

            c. **Naproxen sodium (Aleve)** 550 mg load, then 275 mg q6h.

            d. **Naproxen (Naprosyn)** 500 mg load, then 250 mg q6-8h.

        2. **Oral contraceptives** are also very effective and can be added if the antiprostaglandin is not fully effective.

        3. **Severe dysmenorrhea** that is unresponsive to OC/antiprostaglandin therapy should be evaluated by ultrasonography or laparoscopy.

References, see page 182.

Nocturnal Enuresis

Nocturnal enuresis is defined as the involuntary passage of urine during sleep. Diurnal enuresis refers to the voiding of urine into clothing while awake. Primary nocturnal enuresis is bed wetting that has been present since birth, and secondary nocturnal enuresis is enuresis that occurs after being dry for 6 months. Evaluation of nocturnal enuresis is not necessary unless the problem persists after 4 years of age.

I. **Pathophysiology**
   A. Most bed wetting is due to a maturational delay, and it becomes less frequent with each passing year of life. At age 5, 20% of children wet the bed at least monthly, with 5% of boys and 1% of girls wetting the bed nightly. By age 6, only 10% of children wet the bed. Thereafter, 15% of bed wetters become dry each year. Overall, 60% of bed wetters and more than 90% of nightly bed wetters are male.
   B. **Physiologic enuresis**
      1. Most children who have primary nocturnal enuresis have no disease mechanism to explain the enuresis, and they are considered to have physiologic enuresis. Enuresis results from inability to recognize the sensation of a full bladder during sleep and to awaken from sleep to urinate into the toilet. Those children who wet nightly usually also have a small bladder, which is unable to hold all the urine produced during the night.
      2. Enuresis has a genetic predisposition. If one parent was a bed wetter, the probability of offspring having enuresis is 45%. If both parents were bed wetters, the probability of enuresis is 77%.

II. **Evaluation of nocturnal enuresis**
   A. **History for organic factors**
      1. **Symptoms** of dysuria, intermittent daytime wetness, polydipsia, polyuria, CNS trauma, constipation, and encopresis may indicate medically treatable conditions.
      2. Constant wetness or dampness (ectopic ureter), an abnormal urine with dribbling or hesitancy (posterior urethral valves), or a change in gait (spinal tumor) may indicate surgically treatable conditions.
   B. **Physical examination**
      1. **Abdominal examination** may reveal a distended bladder or fecal impaction. Examination of the lumbosacral area may reveal a midline defect. Gait, muscle tone, strength, and deep tendon reflexes in the lower extremities should be assessed.
      2. **External genitalia** should be examined for meatitis, vulvitis, labial adhesions, or signs of sexual abuse.
      3. If the urine stream is abnormal by history, it should be observed. Rectal examination should be performed if encopresis or constipation is reported.
      4. The dorsum of the feet should be examined for pitting edema. The patient should be examined for obligatory mouth breathing because such children may wet themselves during sleep apnea and be cured by adenoidectomy.
   C. **Laboratory tests.** Every child who has enuresis should have a urinalysis. Absence of glucose rules out diabetes. A specific gravity of 1.015 or greater rules out diabetes insipidus. A urine culture should be obtained if symptoms of

UTI are present, the urine has a foul odor, a nitrite or leukocyte esterase dipstick test is positive, or the patient has had a UTI in the past.

D. **Confirmation of physiologic enuresis**
   1. More than 97% of children do not have a physical cause for their nocturnal enuresis.
   2. **Functional bladder capacity.** The parents should measure functional bladder capacity at least three times before the initial physician evaluation. If this step has not been done, have the child drink 12 oz of water upon arrival for evaluation and measure the volume of urine when the child reports the need to urinate. The normal bladder capacity in ounces is the age plus 2. Normal adult bladder capacity is 12 to 16 oz. If the bladder capacity is normal, the problem usually responds to simple motivational techniques. If bladder capacity is smaller than normal, treatment is more difficult.

Evaluation of Physiologic Enuresis

Bed-wetting status
- Dry nights/month
- Most consecutive dry nights
- Frequency of urination (bladder size)
- Urgency of urination
- Evening fluid intake
- Bladder emptied at bedtime

Awakening to use toilet during the night
- Self-awakens to full bladder
- Self-awakens to wetness
- Never awakens spontaneously
- Awakened by parent
- Evidence for deep sleep, sleepwalking
- Family history of bed wetting or small bladders
- Functional bladder capacity measurement

III. **Nondrug management of nocturnal enuresis**
   A. The parents should be reassured that bed wetting is due to a maturational delay and that it is not intentional. They should be warned about the inappropriateness of any punishment, which can cause psychological scars.
   B. **Getting up at night** can compensate for a small bladder. No child can be cured completely until he learns how to awaken spontaneously, locate the toilet, and urinate there. Nondrug management should include the following:
      1. **Improve access to the toilet.** Put a nightlight in the bathroom. If the bathroom is at a distant location, put a portable toilet in the child's bedroom.
      2. **Avoid excessive fluids two hours before bedtime.** Caffeine-containing beverages should be eliminated. Fluid restrictions should be elected by the child, not imposed.
      3. **Empty the bladder at bedtime.** The parents may need to remind the child.
      4. **Take the child out of diapers or pull-ups.** These items can interfere with motivation for getting up at night.
      5. **Include the child in morning cleanup.** The child should help in stripping the bedclothes and putting them into the washing machine.
      6. **Preserve self-esteem.** Support, encouragement, and an understanding

that the problem is due to a small bladder are important.

C. Self-awakening or parent-awakening programs

1. **Self-awakening.** Ask children to rehearse the going to the bathroom sequence every night before going to sleep. The child lies in bed with eyes closed and pretends that it is the middle of the night and the full bladder is trying to wake him up by starting to hurt. He then goes to the bathroom.

2. **Parent-awakening** is indicated if self-awakening fails. The child should be awakened at the parents' bedtime each night and told to use the bathroom.

D. Enuresis alarms

1. Small alarms that are worn on the body are available to help teach children to awaken to the sensation of a full bladder. Most of them are audio alarms (eg, Nytone or Wetstop). One alarm (The Potty Pager) is a vibrating alarm.

2. Enuresis alarms have the highest cure rate of any treatment, with a 84% cure rate.

IV. Drug therapy

A. Desmopressin

1. Desmopressin (DDAVP), the synthetic analog of vasopressin, reduces urine production by increasing water retention. The drug is administered intranasally. The starting dosage for all ages is one spray in each nostril at bedtime. The dosage can be increased by 10 mcg weekly to a maximum total dose of 40 mcg if the patient is unresponsive.

2. Twenty-four percent of children are completely dry while on medication, and 94.3% relapse after desmopressin is discontinued.

3. Desmopressin costs about $1.50 per spray.

B. Imipramine (Tofranil)

1. Imipramine combines an anticholinergic effect that increases bladder capacity. Imipramine is taken 1 hour before bedtime. The starting dosage is usually 25 mg per day. The maximum dosage is 50 mg/day for children from 8 to 12 years of age and 75 mg/day for children older than 12. Initial cure rates are 10-60%. Relapse rates are 90%.

2. Imipramine should be avoided in children younger than 5 years of age because overdose is often fatal in this age group.

Drugs for Nocturnal Enuresis		
	Desmopressin	**Imipramine**
How supplied	5 mL spray bottle (delivers 10 mcg/spray)	25 mg tablets
Dosage	2 sprays hs. Increase by 1 spray weekly to maximum of 4 sprays/night	8-12 yr: 25-50 mg hs >12 yr: 50-75 mg hs
Cautions	Avoid excessive fluids to prevent hyponatremia	Overdose can be lethal

Drugs for Nocturnal Enuresis		
	Desmopressin	**Imipramine**
Tapering	By 1 spray q 2 wk	By 25 mg q 2 wk
Enuresis alarm	Use simultaneously	Use simultaneously

C. **Drug therapy**
   1. Desmopressin and imipramine have similar efficacy. Imipramine has the advantage of lower cost and ease of administration; desmopressin has the advantage of minimal side effects. Combination of the two may be useful for children who do not respond to either drug alone.
   2. **Intermittent use of drugs** is appropriate for children older than age 8 who need them for special occasions.
   3. **Combination drug and enuresis alarm therapy** is especially helpful for older children who have nightly enuresis.
   4. Untreated bed wetting gradually resolves with time, with a 15% spontaneous cure each year.

References, see page 182.

Poisoning

Poisoning is defined as exposure to an agent that can cause organ dysfunction, leading to injury or death. Children less than 6 years of age account for 60.8% of poisonings.

I. **Clinical evaluation of poisoning**
   A. **The type of toxin** involved should be determined. The time of the exposure and how much time has elapsed should be assessed.

Poisonings Among Children Under 6 Years Old	
Toxin	**Percentage**
Pharmaceuticals	
Analgesics	21.4
Cough/cold preparations	17.3
Topical agents	1.9
Antimicrobials	8.5
Vitamins	8.0
Gastrointestinal preparations	7.0
Hormones	4.2

Toxin	Percentage
Minerals/diuretics	3.2
Antihistamines	3.1
Psychopharmaceuticals	2.7
Cardiovascular drugs	2.5
EENT preparations	2.1
Asthma medications	1.8
Stimulants/street drugs	1.0
Non-pharmaceuticals	
Cleaning products/polishes/deodorizers	20.9
Cosmetics/grooming	19.2
Plants/mushrooms/tobacco	16.1
Foreign body/battery/toys	7.8
Pesticides/herbicides/fungicides	7.4
Chemicals	5.3
Hydrocarbons	4.9
Arts/crafts	3.8
Paints/strippers/adhesives/glues	3.8
Alcohols	3.0
Bites/envenomations	2.1
Food poisoning	2.1

B. **The dose of the toxin** should be assumed to be the maximum amount consistent with the circumstances of the poisoning.

C. **Munchausen syndrome by proxy**

  1. Chemical child abuse should be suspected when childhood poisonings are associated with an insidious and/or inexplicable presentation (eg, recurrent acidosis, polymicrobial sepsis, recurrent malabsorption syndrome, factitious hypoglycemia, failure to thrive).

  2. The syndrome is referred to as "Munchausen syndrome by proxy" when the abuse is perpetrated by a caretaker. Agents may include aspirin, codeine, ethylene glycol, fecal material, insulin, ipecac, laxatives, phenothiazines, table salt, and vitamin A.

II. Physical examination

   A. The first priority in a severely poisoned child is to maintain an airway, ventilation, and circulation.
   B. The vital signs, breath odors, skin, gastrointestinal, cardiovascular, respiratory, and neurologic systems should be assessed.

Physical Findings Associated with Specific Drugs and Chemicals	
Symptom or Sign	**Agents**
Fever	Amphetamines, anticholinergics, antihistamines, aspirin, cocaine, iron, phencyclidine, phenothiazines, phenylpropanolamine, thyroid, tricyclic antidepressants
Hypothermia	Barbiturates, carbamazepine, ethanol, isopropanol, narcotics, phenothiazines
Breath odors: 　Mothballs 　Fruity 　Garlic 　Bitter almond 　Peanuts	 Naphthalene, paradichlorobenzene Isopropanol, acetone, nail polish remover Arsenic, organophosphates Cyanide N-3-pyridylmethyl-N-4-nitrophenylurea (VACOR rat poison)
Hypertension	Amphetamines, cocaine, ephedrine, ergotism, norepinephrine, phenylpropanolamine, tricyclic antidepressants (early)
Hypotension	Antihypertensives, arsenic, barbiturates, benzodiazepines, beta blockers, calcium channel blockers, carbon monoxide, cyanide, disulfiram, iron, nitrites, opiates, phenothiazines, tricyclic antidepressants (late)
Tachypnea	Amphetamine, cocaine, carbon monoxide, cyanide, iron, nicotine, phencyclidine, salicylates
Hypoventilation	Alcohols, anesthetics, barbiturates, benzodiazepines, botulism, chlorinated hydrocarbons, cholinesterase-inhibiting pesticides, cyclic antidepressants, narcotics, nicotine, paralytic shellfish poisoning, solvents, strychnine
Coma	Alcohols, anticonvulsants, barbiturates, benzodiazepines, carbon monoxide, chloral hydrate, cyanide, cyclic antidepressants, hydrocarbons, hypoglycemics, insulin, lithium, narcotics, phenothiazines, salicylates, sedative-hypnotics, solvents
Seizures	Amphetamines, camphor, carbon monoxide, cocaine, gyromitra mushrooms, isoniazid, lead, lindane, nicotine, pesticides, phencyclidine, propoxyphene, salicylates, strychnine, theophylline, tricyclic antidepressants
Miosis	Narcotics, organophosphates, phenothiazines, phencyclidine
Mydriasis	Amphetamine, anticholinergics, antihistamines, atropine, cocaine, phenylpropanolamine, tricyclic antidepressants

Symptom or Sign	Agents
Nystagmus	Phencyclidine, phenytoin
Peripheral neuropathy	Acrylamide, carbon disulfide, heavy metals

C. **Skin examination**
   1. Cyanosis suggests hypoxia secondary to aspiration (eg, hydrocarbon) or asphyxia (eg, apnea due to central nervous system depressants).
   2. The adolescent substance abuser may have needle tracks along veins or scars from subcutaneous injections. Urticaria suggests an allergic reaction. Jaundice may signify hemolysis from naphthalene mothballs.

D. **Cardiovascular effects**
   1. Sympathetic stimulation can cause hypertension with tachycardia.
   2. Hypotension is caused by beta adrenergic blockade, calcium channel blockade, sympatholytic agents, cellular toxins, psychopharmaceutical agents, disulfiram-ethanol, and shock associated with iron or arsenic.

E. **Respiratory effects**
   1. **Tachypnea and hyperpnea** may result from salicylate poisoning. Nervous system stimulants may be associated with tachypnea. Cellular poisons will increase the respiratory rate.
   2. **Central nervous system depressants** may depress the respiratory drive.
   3. **Apnea** may be associated with toxins causing weakness of respiratory muscles. The respiratory examination may reveal poisoning-associated wheezing (eg, beta blocker overdose or inhalants) or crackles (aspiration pneumonia, pulmonary edema).

F. **Neurologic examination**
   1. **Depressed consciousness**, confusion, delirium, or coma may result from toxins, such as ethanol. Central nervous system stimulants or neurotransmitter antagonists produce seizures.
   2. **Pupils.** Dilated pupils can be caused by sympathetic stimulation (eg, amphetamine, cocaine). Constricted pupils are caused by parasympathetics stimulation (eg, organophosphate pesticides) or sympathetic blockade (eg, phenothiazines).
   3. **Sensorimotor examination** may reveal peripheral anesthesia caused solvents, pesticides, or acrylamide.
   4. **Neurologic signs of substance abuse**
      a. **Ethanol, isopropyl alcohol, ethylene glycol, or methanol** can cause an alcoholic state of intoxication. Amphetamine or cocaine often cause agitation, euphoria, or paranoia. Lysergic acid diethylamide (LSD), mescaline, or amphetamine congeners (eg, methylene dioxyamphetamine, MDA) can cause visual or auditory hallucinations.
      b. **Benzodiazepines and narcotics** (oxycodone) can cause drowsiness, slurred speech, confusion, or coma. Phencyclidine (PCP) causes agitation, dissociative delusional thinking, rhabdomyolysis, and a rotatory nystagmus. Glue or gasoline sniffing can result in exhilaration, grandiose delusions, irrational behavior, and sudden death from cardiac dysrhythmias.

III. Laboratory assessment
A. Toxic screens
1. The history and physical examination will usually provide enough information to make a diagnosis and begin therapy. Occasionally, toxin screening of blood and/or urine can confirm the diagnosis.
2. A toxic screen of the blood and urine may include assays for acetone, acetaminophen, amphetamines, anticonvulsants, antidepressants, antihistamines, benzodiazepines, ethanol, isopropanol, methanol, narcotics, neuroleptics, or phencyclidine.

B. Serum osmolarity
1. **The osmolar gap** is derived from the measured serum osmolality minus the calculated serum osmolality (2 x Na + BUN/2.8 + glucose/18). When exogenous osmoles are present (eg, ethanol, isopropyl alcohol, methanol, acetone, or ethylene glycol), the osmolar gap will be elevated.
2. **Anion gap acidosis**
   a. Lactic acid (eg, in ethanol, isoniazid, iron poisonings), ketoacids (eg, diabetes, ethanol), or exogenous organic acids may cause a metabolic acidosis.
   b. Metabolic acidoses are classified as either increased anion gap ([Na+ K] - [Cl + HCO3]) above 15 mEq/L (ethylene glycol, iron, isoniazid, methanol, or salicylate), or depressed anion gap (lithium), or normal anion gap (laxatives, colchicine).

C. Other frequently ordered tests
1. **Hepatic and renal function** should be monitored because most toxins are detoxified in the liver and/or excreted in the urine. Many poisonings are accompanied by rhabdomyolysis (elevated creatinine phosphokinase levels) from seizures, hyperthermia, or muscle spasms.
2. **Urine that fluoresces under Wood lamp** examination is diagnostic of antifreeze poisoning.
3. **Chest and abdominal radiographs** may show radiopacities from calcium tablets, chloral hydrate, foreign bodies, iodine tablets, phenothiazine and antidepressant tablets, and enteric-coated capsules.
4. **Serial electrocardiograms** are essential with antiarrhythmic drugs, beta blockers, calcium channel blockers, lithium, phenothiazines, theophylline, or tricyclic antidepressants.

IV. Toxidromes

Common Toxidromes	
Toxin (Toxidrome)	**Symptoms and Signs**
Abstinence (narcotic withdrawal)	Shivering, nausea, vomiting, diarrhea, abdominal pain, lacrimation, diaphoresis, rhinorrhea, mydriasis, tremor, irritability, lethargy, yawning, delirium, seizures
Anticholinergic	Fever, flushing, dry skin, mydriasis, dry mouth, delirium

Toxin (Toxidrome)	Symptoms and Signs
Cholinergic	Salivation, lacrimation, sweating, bronchorrhea, emesis, incontinence, diarrhea, miosis, muscle weakness, seizures, coma, fasciculation, myoclonus, wheezing, respiratory failure, bradycardia
Iron	Shock, fever, hyperglycemia, hemorrhagic diarrhea
Isoniazid	Seizures, coma, acidosis
Opiates	Coma, respiratory failure, pinpoint pupils
Phenothiazines	Dystonia syndrome, oculogyric crisis, hyperthermia syndrome, coma, prolonged QTc interval
Phencyclidine	Catatonia, rotatory nystagmus, seizures, aggressive paranoia
Salicylates	Fever, hyperpnea, tachypnea, tinnitus, acidosis, seizures
Tricyclic antidepressants	Seizures, coma, acidosis, tachyarrhythmia, prolonged QRS interval, hypotension

V. Diagnostic trials
   A. For a few poisons, a "diagnostic trial" of an antidote can implicate an agent as the cause of a poisoning.

Diagnostic Trials

Toxin	Diagnostic Trial	Route	Positive Response
Benzodiazepine	Flumazenil 0.02 mg/kg	IV	Consciousness improves
Digitalis	Specific Fab antibodies	IV	Dysrhythmia resolves, hyperkalemia improves, consciousness improves
Insulin	Glucose 1 g/kg	IV	Consciousness improves
Iron	Deferoxamine 40 mg/kg	IM	Pink "vin rose" urine
Isoniazid	Pyridoxine 5 g	IV	Seizures abate

Toxin	Diagnostic Trial	Route	Positive Response
Opiate	Naloxone 0.1 mg/kg	IV	Consciousness improves
Phenothi-azine	Diphenhydramine 1 mg/kg	IV	Dystonia and torticollis resolve

VI. Management

A. **Poison centers** can help with the diagnosis and management of poisonings, and assist in locating exotic antidotes.

B. **Initial management of poisoning** involves maintaining an airway, providing ventilatory support, securing vascular access, and initiating resuscitation.

C. **Decontamination**

1. **Skin, mucous membrane, or eye exposures** should be washed with a stream of lukewarm water for 15 to 20 minutes. Soap is used to decontaminate skin exposures.

2. **Emesis** is most effective when less than 1 hour has elapsed since the ingestion; it can remove up to 30% of a toxin in the stomach. Induction of emesis at home may be accomplished with syrup of ipecac. Ipecac is not recommended in infants less than 9 months old. Ipecac is contraindicated in the child who is drowsy or comatose or when the child has ingested a caustic agent or hydrocarbon.

3. **Gastric lavage**

   a. **Decontamination** by lavage is preferred over emesis in the emergency department because it is controllable. Contraindications include nontoxic ingestions, ingestions in which the substance is already past the stomach or absorbed, and caustic or hydrocarbon ingestions.

   b. It is most successful when performed within 90 minutes of the ingestion. For toxins associated with delayed gastric emptying (eg, aspirin, iron, antidepressants, antipsychotics) or for those that can form concretions (eg, iron, salicylates), lavage may be beneficial hours later.

   c. A large-bore (24-32F) orogastric tube is used, and 100- to 200-cc aliquots of warm, normal saline are infused/withdrawn until no more pill fragments are detectable in the lavage fluid or until about 2 liters have been exchanged.

   d. **Activated charcoal** is effective for absorbing most drugs, but it is ineffective for alcohols, caustics, cyanide, heavy metals, lithium, and some pesticides.

   e. Overdoses of carbamazepine, tricyclic antidepressants, and procainamide are managed with multiple doses of charcoal. Contraindications to charcoal include a poisoning where esophageal endoscopy is contemplated, one in which the toxin is not adsorbed by charcoal, or a poisoning in which the patient has an ileus, gastrointestinal hemorrhage, or repeated retching.

4. **Enhanced elimination**

   a. Multiple doses of charcoal also can enhance elimination by "gastrointestinal dialysis." Repetitive doses of charcoal are recommended for phenobarbital, salicylate, and theophylline poisoning.

   b. A cathartic such as magnesium citrate is recommended when charcoal is used because charcoal is constipating. Hemodialysis or hemoperfusion can be life-saving for severe intoxications.

D. Antidotes

Childhood Antidotes	
Toxin	**Antidote**
Acetaminophen	N-Acetylcysteine
Arsenic	BAL, Penicillamine
Benzodiazepine	Flumazenil
Carbon monoxide	Hyperbaric oxygen
Coumadin	Vitamin K1
Cyanide	Sodium nitrite/thiosulfate
Digitalis	Specific Fab antibody fragments
Ethylene glycol/methanol	Ethanol (4-methylpyrazole)
Heparin	Protamine sulfate
Iron	Deferoxamine
Isoniazid	Pyridoxine
Lead	EDTA, Penicillamine, BAL, DMSA
Mercury	BAL
Narcotics	Naloxone
Organophosphate pesticides	Atropine/pralidoxime
Phenothiazines	Diphenhydramine

VII. Specific toxins
A. Acetaminophen (APAP)
1. Single overdoses of greater than 150 mg/kg can cause liver failure. Nausea and abdominal pain are common. The patient may vomit repeatedly, be mildly lethargic, or remain asymptomatic. At 24 to 36 hours after the ingestion, abdominal tenderness and rising serum transaminase levels signify onset of hepatitis that peaks in severity by 96 hours.
2. Acetaminophen exerts its toxic effects is through its hepatic metabolism via cytochrome P450, using glutathione as a cofactor. In an overdose, glutathione is depleted and hepatocytes are damaged.
3. The Rumack nomogram predicts the likelihood of hepatitis. The peak

concentration is measured 4 hours after the ingestion; levels greater than 200 mcg/mL at 4 hours are associated with liver toxicity.
4. When acetaminophen has been taken in high dose, or when acetaminophen levels are in the range likely to cause hepatotoxicity, N-acetylcysteine (NAC) is given at a loading dose of 140 mg/kg, followed by 17 doses of 70 mg/kg separated by 4-hour intervals.
5. Once NAC has been started because of one toxic level, the full course should be given; there is no need to get repeated APAP concentrations.

B. **Alcohols**
1. Alcohols include ethanol, ethylene glycol, methanol, and isopropyl alcohol.
2. Antifreeze contains ethylene glycol, Sterno and windshield wiper fluid contain methanol, jewelry cleaners and rubbing alcohol contain isopropanol.
3. All of the alcohols cause inebriation, loss of motor control and coma. Ethylene glycol may cause acidosis, renal failure, and seizures. Methanol may cause metabolic acidosis, seizures, and blindness. Isopropyl alcohol can produce gastritis, ketosis, and hypotension.
4. Concentrations of ethylene glycol or methanol >20 mg/dL require the use of ethanol therapy to block alcohol dehydrogenase conversion to the toxic metabolites; hemodialysis is indicated for concentrations >50 mg/dL. Isopropanol or ethanol intoxications usually require only close monitoring with frequent measurements of serum glucose. Respiratory depression, seizures, and coma from ethanol poisoning and levels >300-400 mg/dL require hemodialysis.

C. **Caustics**
1. **Drain cleaners** contain sodium hydroxide or sulfuric acid; toilet cleaners may contain hydrochloric or sulfuric acids.
2. **Laundry or dishwasher detergents** may contain sodium metasilicate or sodium triphosphate.
3. **Signs of caustic ingestion** include lip or tongue swelling; burning pain; dysphagia; drooling; and whitish or red plaques on the tongue, buccal or palatal mucosa, or in the perioral area. Caustics can cause severe burns to the esophagus or stomach even in the absence of symptoms.
4. **Inhalations** are managed with humidified oxygen. Skin exposures are washed carefully with soap and water and then treated like any other burn.
5. **Strongly alkaline agents** damage the upper esophagus. **Hydrochloric, sulfuric (muriatic), and other acids** damage the lower esophagus and stomach.
6. **Treatment of caustic ingestions.** The child should be given nothing by mouth, and endoscopic evaluation should be performed 12 to 24 hours after the ingestion. Emesis, lavage and charcoal are contraindicated.

D. **Foreign body ingestion**
1. **Aspirated objects** will cause symptoms of choking, gasping, coughing, cyanosis, wheezing, fever, and poor air entry. While chest radiography can confirm the diagnosis, a negative film does not rule out aspiration. A foreign body requires immediate removal by bronchoscopy.
2. **Ingestion of disc batteries** requires removal when lodged in the esophagus; those in the stomach or beyond should be followed with repeated abdominal films every 2 to 3 days to ensure passage. Disc batteries that have remained in one position for more than 7 days may require surgical removal. Coins or other foreign bodies past the esophagus can be managed with serial radiographs and parental vigilance for their passage.

E. **Hydrocarbons**
1. **Aliphatic hydrocarbons** include kerosene, mineral oil, gasoline, and petrolatum. Kerosene and gasoline are capable of causing an aspiration pneumonia and CNS depression. Petrolatum, mineral oil and motor oil do not carry significant risk of injury. Aliphatic hydrocarbons in small doses are not harmful if left in the stomach. Emesis is contraindicated because of the risk of aspiration; decontamination should be attempted only if a very large dose was taken.
2. **Aromatic hydrocarbons**, such as xylene or toluene, are toxic. Aromatic hydrocarbon ingestions necessitate lavage because of their potent toxicities.
3. **Aspiration pneumonia** is suggested by gasping, choking, coughing, chest pain, dyspnea, cyanosis, leukocytosis, and fever. A chest radiograph may not be diagnostic until hours after ingestion.

F. **Iron**
1. Iron is present in many children's multivitamins, although the worst cases of iron poisoning usually involve prenatal vitamins, which contain 60 mg of elemental iron per tablet. In overdose, iron is a metabolic poison and is corrosive to gastric mucosa, resulting in shock.
2. Ferrous sulfate is 20% elemental iron, ferrous fumarate 33%, and ferrous gluconate 11%. Little toxicity is seen at a dose of elemental iron less than 20 mg/kg. Mild symptoms of poisoning are seen at doses of 20-60 mg/kg; moderate-to-severe symptoms at doses of 60 to 100 mg/kg; life-threatening symptoms at doses greater than 100 mg/kg; and a lethal dose is 180 to 300 mg/kg.
3. **Early symptoms** include nausea, vomiting, fever, hemorrhagic diarrhea, tachycardia, hypotension, hyperglycemia, and acidosis. Intermediate symptoms (8 to 48 hours after ingestion) may include obtundation, coma, fulminant hepatitis, hypoglycemia, clotting abnormalities, pulmonary edema, and renal tubular dysfunction.
4. **Laboratory findings** include a metabolic acidosis with a high anion gap, an abdominal radiograph showing radiopaque pills in the stomach, an elevated white blood cell count greater than 15,000/mm³, and an elevated blood glucose >150 mg/dL. A serum iron concentration, obtained 4 hours after the ingestion, of less than 300 mcg/dL is not toxic; 300 to 500 mcg/dL is mildly toxic, 500 to 1000 mcg/dL is moderately to severely toxic; greater than 1000 mcg/dL is life-threatening.
5. **Treatment.** Decontamination by lavage should be initiated; charcoal is not effective. Volume expansion with intravenous fluids, correction of electrolyte/acid-base disturbances, and intravenous deferoxamine.

G. **Salicylates**
1. Aspirin overdoses greater than 150 mg/kg are toxic. Salicylates are locally corrosive, and tablets can form bezoars near the gastric outlet. Salicylates stimulate the central respiratory center, so that the metabolic acidosis is compensated by a respiratory alkalosis.
2. **Early symptoms** of toxicity include gastrointestinal pain, nausea, vomiting, tinnitus, confusion, lethargy, and fever. Respirations often are rapid and deep. Severe poisonings can be associated with seizures, coma, and respiratory and cardiovascular failure.
3. **Laboratory findings** include hypocalcemia, hypomagnesemia, hypokalemia, and hyperglycemia (early) or hypoglycemia (late).
4. **Serum aspirin concentration** obtained 2 and 6 hours after the ingestion higher than 30 mg/dL are considered toxic, those greater than 70 mg/dL

are associated with severe symptoms, and those greater than 100 mg/dL are life-threatening.

5. **Management** includes lavage, which may be effective as long as 4 to 6 hours after the ingestion. Multiple-dose activated charcoal is effective. Correction of acidemia, hypokalemia, and hypocalcemia are important. Hemodialysis is indicated for serum concentrations greater than 100 mg/dL.

References, see page 182.

Developmental Pediatrics

Infant Growth and Development

Infancy consists of the period from birth to about two years of age. Advances occur in physical growth, motor development, cognitive development, and psychosocial development.

I. **Physical growth milestones**
   A. Fetal weight gain is greatest during the third trimester. Birth weight is regained by 2 weeks of age and doubles by 5 months. During the first few months of life, this rapid growth continues, after which the growth rate decelerates.
   B. Height does not double until between 3 and 4 years of age.
   C. Head growth during the first 5 or 6 months results from continued neuronal cell division. Later, increasing head size is the result of neuronal cell growth and supporting tissue proliferation.
   D. Attainment of growth milestones will vary depending on each child's genetic and ethnic characteristics.

Average Physical Growth Parameters				
Age	**Head circumference**	**Height**	**Weight**	**Dentition**
Birth	35.0 cm (13.8 in) +2 cm/mo (0 to 3 mo) +1 cm/mo (3 to 6 mo) +0.5 cm/mo (6 to 12 mo) Mean = 1 cm/mo	50.8 cm (20.0 in)	3.0 to 3.5 kg (6.6 to 7.7 lb) Regains birthweight by 2 wk Doubles birthweight by 5 mo	Central incisors--6 mo Lateral incisors--8 mo
1 year	47.0 cm (18.5 in)	76.2 cm (30.0 in)	10.0 kg (22 lb) Triples birth-weight	First molars--14 mo Canines--19 mo
2 years	49.0 cm (19.3 in)	88.9 cm (35.0 in)	12.0 to 12.5 kg (26.4 to 27.5 lb) Quadruples birthweight	Second molars--24 mo

   E. **Occipitofrontal circumference**
      1. **Microcephaly** is associated with an increased incidence of mental retardation, but there is no direct relationship between small head size and decreased intelligence. Microcephaly associated with genetic or acquired disorders usually has cognitive implications.

    2. **Macrocephaly** may be caused by hydrocephalus, which is associated with learning disabilities. Macrocephaly without hydrocephalus is associated with cognitive deficits caused by metabolic or anatomic abnormalities. Fifty percent of cases of macrocephaly are familial and have no effect on intellect. When evaluating the infant with macrocephaly, the finding of a large head size in one or both parents is reassuring.

F. Height and weight
1. Although the majority of individuals who are of below- or above-average size are otherwise normal, there is an increased prevalence of developmental disabilities in these two groups.
2. Many genetic syndromes are associated with short stature; large stature syndromes are less common. When considering deviation from the norm, short stature in the family is reassuring.

G. Dysmorphism. Most isolated minor dysmorphic features are inconsequential; however, the presence of three or more indicative of developmental dysfunction. Seventy-five percent of minor superficial dysmorphisms can be found by examining the face, skin, and hands.

II. Motor development milestones
A. Motor milestones are ascertained from the developmental history and observation. Gross motor development begins with holding head up, rolling and progresses to sitting, and then standing, and ambulating.

B. Fine motor development
1. In the first year of life, the pincer grasp develops. During the second year of life, the infant learns to use objects as tools during play.
2. Reaching becomes more accurate, and objects are initially brought to the mouth for oral exploration. As the pincer grasp and macular vision improve, precise manual exploration replaces oral exploration.

C. Red flags in motor development
1. Persistent listing to one side at 3 months of age often is the earliest indication of neuromotor dysfunction.
2. Spontaneous frog-legs posturing suggests hypotonia/weakness, and scissoring suggests spastic hypertonus. Early rolling (1 to 2 months), pulling directly to a stand at 4 months (instead of to a sit), W-sitting, bunny hopping, and persistent toe walking may indicate spasticity.
3. Hand dominance prior to 18 months of age should prompt the clinician to examine the contralateral upper extremity for weakness associated with a hemiparesis.

III. Cognitive development milestones
A. Language is the single best indicator of intellectual potential; problem-solving skills are the next best measure. Gross motor skills correlate least with cognitive potential; most infants with mental retardation walk on time.

B. Problem-solving skills
1. The 1-year-old child recognizes objects and associates them with their functions. Thus, he begins to use them functionally as "tools" instead of mouthing, banging, and throwing them.
2. Midway through the second year, the child begins to label objects and actions and categorize them, allowing the child to match objects that are the same and later to match an object to its picture.
3. **Object permanence**
    a. Prior to the infant's mastery of object permanence, a person or object that is "out of sight" is "out of mind," and its disappearance does not evoke a reaction. Separation anxiety will occur when a loved one leaves the room.

      b. The child will progress to finding an object that has been hidden under a cloth. A more complex task is locating an object that has been wrapped inside a cloth.

      c. The next skill in this sequence is the ability to locate an object under double layers (eg, a cube is placed under a cup and then the cup is covered with a cloth).

      d. This is followed by the ability to locate an object after serial displacements (an object is hidden under one cover and then changed to another one).

  4. Causality. Initially, the infant accidentally discovers that his actions produce a certain effect. The infant then learns that actions cause consistent effects.

C. Language development

  1. Receptive language skills reflect the ability to understand language. Expressive language skills reflect the ability to make thoughts, ideas, and desires known to others.

  2. Prespeech period (0 to 10 months). Receptive language is characterized by an increasing ability to localize sounds, such as a bell. Expressive language consists of cooing. At 3 months, the infant will begin vocalizing after hearing an adult speak. At 6 months of age, the infant adds consonants to the vowel sounds in a repetitive fashion (babbling). When a random vocalization (eg, "dada") is interpreted by the parents as a real word, the parent will show pleasure and joy. In so doing, parents reinforce the repeated use of these sounds.

  3. Naming period (10 to 18 months). The infant's realizes that people have names and objects have labels. The infant begins to use the words "dada" and "mama" appropriately. Infants next recognize and understand their own names and the meaning of "no." By 12 months of age, some infants understand as many as 100 words. They can follow a simple command as long as the speaker uses a gesture. Early in the second year, a gesture no longer is needed.

  4. The infant will say at least one "real" word (ie, other than mama, dada) before his first birthday. At this time, the infant also will begin to verbalize with sentence-like intonation and rhythm (immature jargoning). As expressive vocabulary increases, real words are added (mature jargoning). By 18 months, the infant will use about 25 words.

  5. Word combination period (18 to 24 months). Children begin to combine words 6 to 8 months after they say their first word. Early word combinations are "telegraphic" (eg, "Go out"). A stranger should be able to understand at least 50% of the infant's speech.

D. Red flags in cognitive development

  1. Language development provides an estimate of verbal intelligence; problem-solving provides an estimate of nonverbal intelligence. If deficiencies are global (ie, skills are delayed in both domains), there is a possibility of mental retardation.

  2. When a discrepancy exists between problem-solving and language abilities, with only language being deficient, the possibility of a hearing impairment or a communication disorder should be excluded.

  3. If either language or problem-solving skills is deficient, the child is at high risk for a learning disability later.

  4. All children who have delayed language development should receive audiologic testing to rule out hearing loss. Deaf infants will begin to babble on time at 6 months, but these vocalizations will gradually decline thereafter.

IV. Psychosocial development
  A. **Emotional development**. Emotions are present in infancy and motivate expression (pain elicits crying). Emotions are mediated through the limbic system.
  B. **Social development**
    1. Social milestones begin with bonding, which reflects the feeling of the caregiver for the child. Attachment represents the feeling of the infant for the caregiver, and it develops within a few months.
    2. When recognition of and attachment to a caregiver develops, the simple sight of this person will elicit a smile. The infant becomes more discriminating in producing a smile as he begins to differentiate between familiar and unfamiliar faces. The infant learns to use smiling to manipulate the environment and satisfy personal needs.
    3. Temperament represents the style of a child's emotional and behavioral response to situations.
  C. **Adaptive skill development.** Adaptive skills consist of the skills required for independence in feeding, dressing, toileting, and other activities of daily living. Development of adaptive skill is influenced by the infant's social environment, and by motor and cognitive skill attainment.
  D. **Red flags in psychosocial development**
    1. **Colic** may be an early indication of a "difficult" temperament.
    2. **Delay in the appearance of a smile** suggests an attachment problem, which may be associated with maternal depression. In severe cases, child neglect or abuse may be suspected. A delay in smiling also may be caused by visual or cognitive impairment.
    3. **Failure to develop social relationships** suggests autism when it is accompanied by delayed or deviant language development and stereotypic behaviors.
    4. **Delays in adaptive skills** may indicate overprotective parents or an excessive emphasis on cleanliness or orderliness.

References, see page 182.

Toddler Development

Toddlerhood consists of the years from about 1 to 3 years of age. Affective development is highlighted by the toddler's striving for autonomy and independence, attachment to family, and the development of impulse control. Cognitive development is characterized by the transition from sensorimotor to preoperational thought.

I. Growth rate and physical appearance
  A. After the rapid growth of infancy, the rate of growth slows in the toddler years. After age 2, toddlers gain about 5 lb in weight and 2.5 inches in height each year. Growth often occurs in spurts. Between the ages of 2 and 2.5 years, the child will have reached 50% of his adult height.
  B. Growth of the lower extremities often is accompanied by tibial torsion and physiologic bowing of the legs, which usually corrects by age 3 years. The percentage of body fat steadily decreases from 22% at age 1 year to about 15% at age 5 years.

II. Gross motor skills

    A. Most children walk without assistance by 18 months. At 2 years, the stiff, wide-leg gait of early toddlerhood becomes a flexible, steady walking pattern, with heel-toe progression.

Gross Motor Abilities
18 Months
• Walking fast, seldom falling • Running stiffly • Walking up stairs with one hand held • Seating self in a small chair • Climbing into an adult chair • Hurling a ball
24 Months
• Running well without falling • Walking up and down stairs alone • Kicking a large ball
36 Months
• Walking up stairs by alternating feet • Walking well on toes • Pedaling a tricycle • Jumping from a step • Hopping two or three times

III. Fine motor skills

    A. The 18-month-old can make a tower of four blocks. One year later, he can stack eight blocks. Most 18-month-olds will hold the crayon in a fist and scribble spontaneously on paper.

Fine Motor Abilities
18 Months
• Making a tower of four cubes • Releasing 10 cubes into a cup • Scribbling spontaneously • Imitating a vertically drawn line

24 Months
• Building a seven cube tower • Aligning two or more cubes to form a train • Imitating a horizontally drawn line • Beginning circular strokes • Inserting a square block into a square hole

36 Months
• Copying a circle • Copying bridges with cubes • Building a tower of 9 to 10 blocks • Drawing a person's head

IV. **Affective development**
   A. **Autonomy and independence.** Because of improved motor skills, the transition from infancy to toddlerhood is marked increased autonomy and independence. The toddler may refuse to eat unless allowed to feed himself, and the child may no longer may be willing to try new foods.
   B. **Impulse control.** Toddlers begin to develop impulse control. The 18-month-old may have minimal impulse control and display several temper tantrums each day. Most 3-year-olds have some degree of self-control.
   C. **Successful toileting** usually occurs toward the end of the third year when the child becomes able to control his sphincter, undress, get onto the potty, and has the willingness to participate. Success with consistent daytime dryness usually is not achieved until about 2.5 years of age.

Social/Emotional Skills

18 Months
• Removing a garment • Feeding self and spilling food • Hugging a doll • Pulling a toy

24 Months
• Using a spoon; spilling little food • Verbalizing toileting needs • Pulling on a simple garment • Verbalizing immediate experiences • Referring to self by name

---

36 Months

- Showing concern about the actions of others
- Playing cooperatively in small groups
- Developing the beginnings of true friendships
- Playing with imaginary friends

    D. Attachment refers to the bond that forms between the infant and the caregiver. Disorders of attachment may result from inconsistent caregiving and are more common in the presence of poverty, drug use, or emotional illness.

    E. Temperament determines how a child approaches a given situation. Ten percent of children are less adaptable and tend to be emotionally negative and are considered "difficult."

V. Cognitive development

    A. Toddlerhood is characterized by a transition from sensorimotor to preoperational thinking. During the sensorimotor period, the infant primarily learns about the world by touching, looking, and listening. Preoperational thought is marked by the development of symbolic thinking, as the child becomes capable of forming mental images and begins to solve problems. Progression from sensorimotor to symbolic thought occurs typically between 18 and 24 months of age.

    B. Complete object permanence has developed, and the child can find an object under a blanket, despite not seeing it hidden.

    C. By 3 years, he can draw primitive figures that represent people, and he develops elaborate play and imagination.

Intellectual Abilities

18 Months

- Pointing to named body parts
- Understanding of object permanence
- Beginning to understand cause and effect

24 Months

- Forming mental images of objects
- Solving problems by trial and error
- Understanding simple time concepts

36 Months

- Asking "why" questions
- Understanding daily routine
- Appreciating special events, such as birthdays
- Remembering and reciting nursery rhymes
- Repeating three digits

VI. Language

A. Beginning around age 2 years, toddlers use language to convey their thoughts and needs (eg, hunger). The 18-month-old has a vocabulary of at least 20 words, consisting primarily of the names of caregivers, favorite foods, and activities.

B. After 18 months the toddler begins to put together phrases. Early two and three word sentences are referred to as "telegraphic speech," and about 50% of what the child says should be intelligible to strangers.

C. By the age of 3 years, the vocabulary increases to about 500 words, and 75% of speech is understandable to strangers. He begins to make complete sentences, and frequently asks "why" questions.

Language Skills
18 Months
<ul><li>Looking selectively at a book</li><li>Using 10 to 20 words</li><li>Naming and pointing to one picture card</li><li>Naming an object (eg, ball)</li><li>Following two-directional commands</li></ul>
24 Months
<ul><li>Using two to three word sentences</li><li>Using "I," "me," "you"</li><li>Naming three picture cards</li><li>Naming two objects</li><li>Knowing four-directional commands</li></ul>
36 Months
<ul><li>Using four to five word sentences</li><li>Telling stories</li><li>Using plurals</li><li>Recognizing and naming most common objects</li></ul>

References, see page 182.

Preschooler Development

I. Family relationships

A. **Separation**. The average 3-year-old child can separate easily from parents. Some children cope by adopting a transitional object, usually a soft object, which serves as a symbolic reminder of the parent.

B. **Fears and fantasies**. Early fantasy, may be indistinguishable from reality, resulting in a tendency for fears. By the age of 4, children frequently have frightening dreams that they can state are "not real."

C. **Temper tantrums** are characteristic of 2-year-olds, but they should be infrequent by age 5, although there is another peak at 6 years in response to the stresses of schooling. Temper tantrums can be exacerbated by: reinforcement by the parents; modeling in the family; exposure to violence, including physical punishment; temperamental low threshold, high reactivity, or lack of adaptability; fatigue; hunger; and lack of routines. They are worsened by parental over concern and attempts to avoid tantrums through giving in.

D. Oppositionality. Preschool children comply with adult requests about 50% of the time. Parents who are authoritative and firm but also warm, encouraging, and rational are more likely to have children who are self-reliant and self-controlled. A system of discipline should include positive reinforcement for desired behaviors; consequences for undesired behaviors; and interactions that promote the parent-child relationship.

E. Sibling interactions

1. Factors associated with greater sibling rivalry, include opposite gender, difficult temperament, insecure pattern of attachment, family discord, and corporal punishment. Preschool children often "regress" when a new baby is born, exhibiting increased naughtiness, thumb sucking, and altered toileting.

2. Sibling classes, avoidance of forced interactions, a strong pre-existing relationship between the older child and the father, good support for the mother postpartum, individual time continued with each parent, and talking about the new baby are helpful.

3. Interaction between siblings can be improved through prompt limiting of aggression toward the sibling, acknowledgment of the child's feelings, reinforcement through praise, and distraction, trading, taking turns, and teaching.

4. Minor sibling skirmishes should be ignored. During serious disputes, the children or the object of dispute should be removed. Physical battles require a time-out for both children.

II. Peer relationships

A. Play

1. At the age of 2 years, most play is parallel. By the age of 3, children should have mastered aggression and should be able to initiate play with a peer, have joint goals in their play together, and take turns. Fantasy or pretend play gains prominence at about age 3.

2. Pretend friends are very common in children up to the age of 4. Mastery of aggressive impulses should improve after 2½ years of age. Hostile aggression is more common in boys, especially those who have poor impulse control, who are punished physically, who view violence, or who are suffering from a difficult separation experience.

50 Preschooler Development

Peer Relationships

	2-year visit	3-year visit	4-year visit	5-year visit
Amount of interaction	Parallel play with peers, copies others, self-talk, solitary play, offers toy, plays games	Takes on a role, prefers some friends over others, plays associatively with others	Interactive games, best friend <2 y difference, may visit neighbor by self, plays cooperatively with others	Group of friends
Duration of interaction	Briefly alone from adult, sudden shifts in intensity of activity	20 min with peers	Prefers peer play to solitary	
Level of fantasy	Symbolic doll, action figures; mimics domestic activities	Simple fantasy play; unfamiliar may be monsters	Elaborate fantasy play, distinguishes fantasy from reality, tells fanciful tales	Make-believe and dress up
Imaginary friends		May have one	Common	If present, private
Favorite toys/activities	Things that move, turn, or fit together; water; books; music; listens to stories	Listens to stories, dresses and undresses dolls	Sings a song, dances, acts, listens to stories	
Rule use	Able to take turns, beginning property rights, "mine," "right places"	Shares some	Shares spontaneously, follows rules in simple games, facility with rules, alternately demanding/cooperative	Follows rules of the game, follows community rules
Aggression	Aggressive to get things	Negotiates conflicts	Wants to please friends	

Development of Independence

	2-year visit	3-year visit	4-year visit	5-year visit
Eating	Uses utensils	Spills little,	Helps set ta-	Helps cook

	2-year visit	3-year visit	4-year visit	5-year visit
Dressing	Undresses, pulls on simple garment	Dresses with supervision, unbuttons some	Dresses all but tying	
Toileting	Clean and dry, but with adult effort and motivation	Clean and dry by self-motivated approach	Independent	

Motor and Cognitive Play Skills				
	2-year visit	3-year visit	4-year visit	5-year visit
Pencil grip	Point down	Awkward, high		Standard
Drawings Identifies Imitates Copies Person-body parts	Vertical, scribble	Shapes Horizontal, cross Circle before cross 2 parts	Longer line Cross before square 6 parts	Directions Square before triangle 10, including head, body, arms, legs
Scissors	One hand	Across paper	Cuts out square	
Block tower	6-9	Tower of 10		
Block figure	Aligns 4 for train	3 block bridge	5 block gate	Steps
Other	Turns pages 1 at a time			Ties knot in string, prints letters

III. Communication

   A. The 2-year-old has a vocabulary of approximately 150 to 500 words. The child should be speaking in two-word utterances (eg, "my Mommy" or "more milk"). They often mimic what others say exactly in whole or in part (echolalia) up to age 2.5 years. Criterion for referral at 2 years of age is a less than a 50-word vocabulary or not putting two words together.

   B. The 3-year-old speaks in simple sentences of three or four words. Sentence length increases by one or two words annually throughout the preschool period, with at least the same number of words that the child is old. The typical 3-year-old can count three items and a 4-year-old can count four items, although they often can recite more of the numbers. A 4-year-old who cannot converse with familiar people with sentences averaging three words should be evaluated.

C. A 5-year-old should use complete sentences containing five words. The 5-year-old can count ten objects or more and should understand "before," "after," and "until"; "if, then." They can discuss emotions and tell jokes. Preschool children who have expressive language disorders tend to speak less often and convey less information than their peers.

D. Strangers should be able to understand 25% to 50% of what the 2-year-old child says. By 3 years of age, strangers should be able to understand the child 75% of the time. By the age of 4, strangers can understand the child 100% of the time, although errors in "r," "s," "l," "sh," and "th" sounds are not uncommon until age 7.

E. Dysfluency (aberration of speech rate and rhythm) occurs transiently between about 2.5 and 4 years of age. Persistent and worsening stuttering beyond the age of 4 should be evaluated.

Communication Skills in Preschoolers

	2-year visit	3-year visit	4-year visit	5-year visit
Vocabulary	No jargon; 150 to 500 words			Definitions
Sentence length	2 words	3 to 4 words	4 to 5 words	
Intelligibility to stranger	25%	75%	100%	
Grammatic forms	Verbs, some adjectives and adverbs	Plurals, pronouns	Past tense	Future tense
Typical examples	Talks about current action, no jargon, names pictures	Tells own age and sex, counts to 3	Describes recent experiences, can sing songs, gives first and last names, counts to 4, identifies gender	Counts to 10 or more, recognizes letters of the alphabet, knows telephone number and address
Fluency	Dysfluency common	Dysfluency common	Some dysfluency	Dysfuencies not expected

Comprehension

	2-year visit	3-year visit	4-year visit	5-year visit
Number step command	100% for 1 without gesture	2	3	

	2-year visit	3-year visit	4-year visit	5-year visit
Number of body parts	names 1, identifies 7			
Number of colors		2 named	4 named	
Gender		self	self and others	
Own names	refers to self by name	first and last		
Numbers counted	says "2" (not counted)	counts to 3		10, knows number
Relationships		which is bigger, under	which is longer, 2 opposites	

Motor development				
	2-year visit	3-year visit	4-year visit	5-year visit
Walks forward	slightly bent	swings arms	tandem walks	
Walks backward	10 ft			tandem
Runs	changing direction	alternating arms		
Climbs	out of crib (2.5 y)	high equipment		
Jumps	both feet off floor	26 to 30 in from both feet	32 in, one foot leads	over 10 in
Jumps down	step with both feet	16 in, lands on one foot first	18 in, lands on both feet	
Stairs-up	one step at a time	without rail, alternating		
Stairs-down	one step at a time	alternating, no rail	alternating	
Stands on one foot	tries	1 sec on 1 foot	5 to 6 sec on each foot	10 sec

	2-year visit	3-year visit	4-year visit	5-year visit
Kicks	kicks ball 6 ft			
Hops		3 hops in place	5 forward	20 ft forward 10 times
Throws	throws 5 ft	bounce, overhand	10 ft, 1 or 2 arms	
Catches		straight arms	bent arm	bounce pass
Skips				skips
Pedals		10 ft, tricy-cle		

References, see page 182.

Attention-Deficit/Hyperactivity Disorders

Attention-deficit/hyperactivity disorder (AD/HD) affects about 5% of girls and 10% of boys of elementary age. AD/HD can interfere with an individual's ability to inhibit behavior (impulsivity) and/or function efficiently in goal-oriented activities (inattention). Symptoms of AD/HD emerge in early childhood and continue to be present into adulthood in up to 70% of cases.

I. **Clinical evaluation**
   A. Three behavioral subtypes of ADHDs are defined: predominantly inattentive, predominantly hyperactive/impulsive, and combined. The symptoms must be chronic and have persisted for more than 6 months. Some symptoms should be present before age 7.
   B. A comprehensive, developmentally oriented evaluation should assess the child's functioning within academic and psychosocial contexts.
   C. Findings on sensory, physical, and neurologic examinations are usually normal. Motor coordination, language skills, and social style should be assessed. Behavioral observations should be interpreted cautiously because children may show few symptoms of AD/HD in the office setting.
   D. Laboratory studies, such as a thyroid screen or electroencephalography, should be based on clinical indications. Lead levels and hematocrit should be considered in preschool children.

DSM-IV Diagnostic Criteria for Attention-Deficit Hyperactivity Disorder

At least six of the following symptoms of inattention or hyperactivity-impulsivity must be evident:

Inattention
Lack of attention to details or careless mistakes in schoolwork or other activities
Difficulty sustaining attention in tasks or play activities
Impression of not listening when spoken to directly
Failure to follow through on instructions or finish schoolwork or duties
Difficulty organizing tasks and activities
Avoidance or dislike of tasks that require sustained mental effort (eg, school-work or homework)
Tendency to lose things necessary for tasks or activities (eg, toys, school assignments, pencils, books)
Distractions by extraneous stimuli
Forgetfulness in daily activities

Hyperactivity
Fidgeting with hands or feet or squirming in seat
Not remaining seated when expected
Running about or climbing excessively
Difficulty engaging in leisure activities quietly
Often "on the go" or "driven by a motor"
Excessive talking

And/Or

Impulsivity
Tendency to blurt out answers before questions have been completed
Difficulty awaiting turn
Tendency to interrupt or intrude on others (eg, butting into conversations or games)

Exclusionary Criteria
A. Some hyperactive-impulsive or inattentive symptoms that caused impairment must have been present before age 7.
B. Some impairment from the symptoms must be present in two or more settings (eg, at school and at home).
C. There must be clear evidence of clinically significant impairment in social, academic or occupational functioning.
D. The symptoms do not occur exclusively during the course of a pervasive developmental disorder, schizophrenia, or other psychotic disorder, and are not better accounted for by another mental disorder.

II. Management
   A. **Behavioral interventions.** Parents may need training in basic management or behavior modification. The child may benefit from social skills training or cognitive-behavioral therapies.
   B. Behavior modification strategies can be used to decrease less desirable behaviors (eg, hitting), increase more desirable behaviors (eg, using words

instead of actions), or teach a new skill (eg, negotiating). Strategies used to modify the behaviors include increased positive attention (eg, "time-in"), punishment (eg, "time-out"), and "selective ignoring." Charts or point systems that track specific behaviors are useful.

C. Stimulant medications

 1. Methylphenidate is the most commonly used stimulant. Other stimulants include dextro-amphetamine pemoline, and a combination of amphetamine salts (Adderall).

 2. **Effects of stimulants**. Stimulants have significant short-term benefits in at least 70% to 80% of children who have AD/HDs.

 3. **Stimulant side effects**

   a. Behavioral rebound, characterized by increased irritability and activity, may occur as the last dose is wearing off. A small additional dose may be beneficial in the afternoon.

   b. Tics or dyskinesias are an infrequent side effect of stimulants. There is no evidence that stimulants cause permanent tic disorders. About 50% to 60% of children who have Tourette syndrome (TS) also have AD/HD, which often presents 2 to 3 years before the onset of tics.

   c. Appetite suppression is common with stimulant use and may result in transitory effects on weight and decreases in height velocity. There is no evidence of any effect on adolescent growth or ultimate adult height. Appetite suppression often diminishes over time.

Stimulant Medications for AD/HDs			
Medication	**Dose schedule**	**Dose range**	**Potential side effects/cautions**
Methylphenidate (Ritalin or generic) 5-, 10-, 20-mg tablets	Initial: 5 mg or 0.3 mg/kg per dose Increase: 2.5 mg to 5 mg weekly Frequency: 2 to 3 doses/d	5 to 80 mg/d 0.3 to 0.8 mg/kg per dose	Anorexia, insomnia, stomach aches, headaches, irritability, "rebound," flattened affect, social withdrawal, weepiness, tics, weight loss, reduced growth velocity Avoid decongestants Monitor height, weight, blood pressure, pulse
Ritalin SR or generic20-mg sustained-release tablets only	Initial: 20 mg Increase: 20 mg Frequency: 1 or 2 doses/d	20 to 80 mg/d 0.6 to 2 mg/kg per dose	Same as regular MPH. May release unevenly Do not chew or cut in half 20 mg SR may be equivalent to 12 to 15 mg regular released over 5 to 8 h

Dextroamphetamine (Dexedrine) 5-mg tablets (Dextrostat) 5-, 10-mg tablets	Initial: 2.5 to 5 mg (0.15 mg/kg per dose) Increase: 2.5 mg to 5 mg weekly Frequency: 2 to 3 doses/d	2.5 to 40 mg/d 0.15 to 0.4 mg/kg per dose	Anorexia, insomnia, stomach aches, headaches, irritability, "rebound," tics, stereotypy, weight loss/reduced growth velocity Avoid decongestants Monitor height, weight, blood pressure, pulse
Dexedrine Spansules 5-, 10-, 15-mg capsules	Initial: 5 mg in AM (0.3 mg/kg per dose) Increase: 5 mg weekly Frequency: 1 to 2 doses/d	5 to 40 mg/d 0.3 to 0.8 mg/kg per dose	Anorexia, insomnia, stomach aches, headaches, irritability, social withdrawal, weepiness, stereotypy, tics, weight loss, reduced growth velocity Avoid decongestants Monitor height, weight, blood pressure, pulse
Mixed Amphetamine Salts (Adderall) 5, 10, 20, 30 mg	Initial: 2.5 to 5 mg in AM Increase: 2.5 to 5 mg weekly Frequency: 1 to 2 doses/d	2.5 to 40 mg/d	Similar to dextroamphetamine Well tolerated
Pemoline (Cylert) 18.75-, 37.5-, 75-mg tablets 37.5-mg chewable tablets	Initial: 37.5 mg in AM Increase: 18.25 mg weekly Frequency: 1 to 2 doses/d Must be taken daily	18.75 to 112.5 mg/d 2 mg/kg per day	Insomnia, anorexia, stomach aches, irritability, headaches, choreoathetoid movements, liver dysfunction, rare fulminant liver failure Monitor height, weight, blood pressure, pulse Obtain liver function tests at baseline and 2 to 3 times per year

D. Nonstimulant medications

1. Nonstimulant medications may be beneficial in children who respond poorly to an adequate trial of stimulants, experience unacceptable stimulant side effects, or have comorbid conditions (tics, anxiety, mood disorder).

Nonstimulant Medications for AD/HDs		
Medication	**Indications**	**Dose schedule**
Imipramine (Tofranil or generic) 10-, 25-, 50-mg tablets	Alternative to stimulant AD/HD + tics Enuresis Anxiety	Initial: 10 to 25 mg or 0.5 mg/kg bedtime Increase: 10 to 25 mg every 5 to 7 d up to 3 mg/kg per day Frequency: 2 to 3 doses/d Must be taken daily. Stop slowly
Desipramine (Norpramin or generic) 10-, 25-, 50-, 75-mg tablets	Alternative to stimulant AD/HD + tics Anxiety	Initial: 25 mg in morning Increase: 25 mg every 5 to 7 d Frequency: 2 to 3 doses/d Must be taken daily. Stop slowly
Nortriptyline (Pamelor or generic) 10-, 25-, 50-, 75-mg tablets 10 mg/5 mL liquid	Alternative to stimulant AD/HD + tics Anxiety	Initial: 10 to 25 mg at bedtime Increase: Up to 2 mg/kg per day Frequency: Once or twice a day
Bupropion (Wellbutrin) 75, 100 mg (Wellbutrin SR) 100, 150 mg	Alternative to stimulant Mood lability Depression Aggression	Initial: 100 SR QD Increase: 50 mg every 1 to 2 wkFrequency: 2 doses/d Must be taken daily.
Clonidine (Catapres or generic) 0.1-, 0.2-, 0.3-mg tablets	Alternative to stimulant AD/HD + tics Insomnia Oppositionality Hyperarousal Aggression	Initial: 0.05 mg HS Increase: 0.05 mg every 3 to 7 d Frequency: 2 to 4 doses/d for AD/HD Start and stop slowly
Catapres TTS 1, 2, 3 (transdermal patches)	Same as clonidine Sustained delivery avoids multiple dosing Less sedating	Initial: TTS 1 patch (0.1 mg/d) Increase: 0.1 mg in 2 wk Frequency: Change every 5 d Beclomethasone nonaqueous nasal spray applied to site decreases irritation
Guanfacine (Tenex or generic) 1-, 2-mg tablets	Same as clonidine Longer half-life and much less sedation than clonidine	Initial dose: 0.5 mg HS Increase: 0.5 mg/wk Give as one to two doses/d Takes several days to weeks to take effect

2. **Tricyclic antidepressants** (TCAs) are efficacious in 60% to 70% of children who have AD/HDs. Those who have AD/HDs and comorbid anxiety, depression, or tic disorders may respond better to TCAs than to stimulants.

E. **Antihypertensives.** A positive behavioral response to clonidine occurs in up to 50% of patients. The best responders tend to be those who are overaroused, easily frustrated, extremely hyperactive, or aggressive. Clonidine has been used as a first-line treatment in children who have comorbid tics or Tourette's syndrome or as an alternative to stimulants when there are severe side effects. Clonidine is not as effective as stimulants.

References, see page 182.

Failure to Thrive

Failure to thrive (FTT) is usually first considered when a child is found to weigh less than the third percentile for age and gender. Although FTT occurs in all socioeconomic strata, it is more frequent in families living in poverty. FTT describes a sign -- it is not a diagnosis. The underlying etiology must be determined. Ten percent of children seen in the primary care setting show signs of growth failure. Children with FTT attain lower verbal intelligence, poorer language development, less developed reading skills, lower social maturity, and have a higher incidence of behavioral disturbances.

I. **Pathophysiology**
  A. **Diagnostic criteria for failure to thrive**
    1. A child younger than 2 years of age whose weight is below the 3rd or 5th percentile for age on more than one occasion.
    2. A child younger than 2 years of age whose weight is less than 80% of the ideal weight for age.
    3. A child younger than 2 years of age whose weight crosses two major percentiles downward on a standardized growth grid.
  B. **Exceptions** to the previously noted criteria include the following:
    1. Children of genetically short stature.
    2. Small-for-gestational age infants.
    3. Preterm infants.
    4. "Overweight" infants whose rate of height gain increases while the rate of weight gain decreases.
    5. Infants who are normally lean.
  C. Many patients with FTT have either an organic or nonorganic cause; however, a sizable number of patients have both psychosocial and organic causes for their condition. FTT is a syndrome of malnutrition brought on by a combination of organic, behavioral, and environmental factors.
II. **Clinical evaluation of poor weight gain or weight loss**
  A. **Feeding history** should assess details of breast or formula feeding, timing and introduction of solids, who feeds the infant, position and placement of the infant for feeding, and stooling or vomiting patterns.
  B. **Developmental history** should cover gestational and perinatal history, developmental milestones, infant temperament, and the infant's daily routine.
  C. **Psychosocial history** should include family composition, employment status, financial status, stress, isolation, child-rearing beliefs, maternal depression, and the caretaker's own history of possible childhood abuse or neglect.
  D. **Family history** should include heights, weights, illnesses, and constitutional short stature, inherited diseases, or developmental delay.

Causes of Inadequate Caloric Intake

Lack of Appetite
- Anemia (eg, iron deficiency)
- Psychosocial problems (eg, apathy)
- Central nervous system (CNS) pathology (eg, hydrocephalus, tumor)
- Chronic infection (eg, urinary tract infection, acquired immunodeficiency syndrome)
- Gastrointestinal disorder (eg, pain from reflux esophagitis)

Difficulty with Ingestion
- Psychosocial problems (eg, apathy, rumination)
- Cerebral palsy/CNS disorder (eg, hypertonia, hypotonia)
- Craniofacial anomalies (eg, choanal atresia, cleft lip and palate micrognathia, glossoptosis)
- Dyspnea (congenital heart disease, pulmonary disease)
- Feeding disorder
- Generalized muscle weakness/pathology (eg, myopathies)
- Tracheoesophageal fistula
- Genetic syndrome (eg, Smith-Lemli-Opitz-syndrome)
- Congenital syndrome (eg, fetal alcohol syndrome)

Unavailability of Food
- Inappropriate feeding technique
- Inadequate volume of food
- Inappropriate food for age
- Withholding of food (abuse, neglect, psychosocial)

Vomiting
- CNS pathology (increased intracranial pressure)
- Intestinal tract obstruction (eg, pyloric stenosis, malrotation)
- Gastroesophageal reflux
- Drugs (eg, syrup of ipecac)

III. **Physical examination**
   A. **Height, weight, and head circumference** should be plotted on a standard growth curve. Three measurements that are below the 3rd percentile indicate an underlying organic disease. If all three measurements are consistently below the third percentile but show the same rate of increase over a period of time, the infant probably had intrauterine growth retardation. If the child's median age for weight is less than the median age for height, the child may be undernourished.
   B. **Dysmorphic features and physical signs** of central nervous system, pulmonary, cardiac, or gastrointestinal disorders, or signs of neglect or abuse (poor hygiene, unexplained bruises or scars, or inappropriate behavior) should be sought.
   C. **Observation of the infant and caretaker.** While feeding and playing, the infant may avoid eye contact or withdraw from physical attention and may show a poor suck or swallow, or aversion to oral stimulation. Ineffective feeding technique or inappropriate response to the infant's physiologic or social cues may be displayed by the caretaker.

D. Diagnostic testing
    1. Laboratory testing. Tests that will usually exclude an organic pathology include a complete blood count, urinalysis, urine culture, blood urea nitrogen, creatinine, serum electrolyte levels, and a tuberculin test.
    2. Radiologic determination of bone age. If the bone age is normal, it is unlikely that the infant has a systemic chronic disease or a hormonal abnormality as the cause of poor weight gain.
    3. Severe malnutrition requires measurement of albumin, alkaline phosphatase, calcium, and phosphorous to assess protein status and to look for biochemical rickets.
    4. Human immunodeficiency virus screening or a sweat test may be considered.
E. A feeding evaluation by a nutritionist or an occupational therapist may detect a subtle feeding disorder.

Causes of Inadequate Calorie Absorption

Malabsorption
- Biliary atresia or cirrhosis
- Celiac disease
- Cystic fibrosis
- Enzymatic deficiencies
- Food (protein) sensitivity or intolerance
- Immunologic deficiency
- Inflammatory bowel disease

Diarrhea
- Bacterial gastroenteritis
- Parasitic infection

Hepatitis

Hirschsprung Disease

Refeeding diarrhea

Causes of Increased Calorie Requirements

Increased Metabolism/Increased Use of Calories
- Chronic/recurrent infection (eg, urinary tract infection, tuberculosis)
- Chronic respiratory insufficiency (eg, bronchopulmonary dysplasia)
- Congenital heart disease/acquired heart disease
- Malignancy
- Chronic anemia
- Toxins (lead)
- Drugs (eg, excess levothyroxine)
- Endocrine disorders (eg, hyperthyroidism, hyperaldosteronism)

Defective Use of Calories
- Metabolic disorders (eg, aminoacidopathies, inborn errors of carbohydrate metabolism)
- Renal tubular acidosis
- Chronic hypoxemia (eg, cyanotic heart disease)

IV. **Treatment of failure to thrive**
  A. The normal, healthy infant requires an average of 100 kcal/kg of body weight per day. Nutritional requirements in children with FTT usually are 150 kcal/kg per day.
  B. **Treatment of infants**
    1. The number of calories per ounce of formula can be increased by adding less water (13 oz infant formula concentrate mixed with 10 oz water provides 24 kcal/oz high-calorie formula) or by adding more carbohydrate in the form of glucose polymers or fat in the form of medium-chain triglycerides or corn oil.
    2. Once nutritional recovery begins, the infant often demands and eats enough food to gain weight. At this point, ad libitum oral feedings are appropriate.
  C. **Treatment of older children.** Foods can be fortified with such items as milk products, margarine, oil, and peanut butter. For the infant or toddler who does not gain weight despite being offered oral feedings, the diet should be supplemented by nasogastric tube feeding.
  D. **Parental behavioral advice**
    1. Try to relax; feeding/eating and meal times should be pleasant. Avoid battles over eating. Encourage the child, but avoid forced feeding or punitive approaches.
    2. Use positive reinforcement (eg, praise for eating well). The withholding of food is not an appropriate form of punishment.
    3. Accept your child's wish to feed himself. Accept that there will be a mess and be prepared (eg, newspaper on the floor).
    4. Try to eat together as a family. Young children like to mimic the good eating behavior of older siblings and parents.
    5. Allow about 1 hour without food or drink (except water) before a meal to stimulate the appetite.
    6. Offer solids before liquids and limit juices to 4 to 8 ounces per day. Consumption of excessive fluids reduces the intake of solid foods.
    7. Establish a routine of meals and snacks at set times. Avoid snacks right

after an unfinished meal.
8. Recognize your child's cues indicating hunger, satiety, and food prefer-
   ences.
9. Limit possible distractions (eg, television) during meals.

References, see page 182.

Speech and Language Development

Language is defined as a symbolic system for the storage and exchange of information.
Language consists of auditory expressive ability (speech), receptive ability (listening
comprehension), and visual communication (gestures).

I. Normal speech and language development
   A. Auditory expressive language development
      1. **In the first 4 to 6 weeks**, the earliest sounds consist of cooing.
      2. **In the first few months**, bilabial sounds begin, consisting of blowing
         bubbles or the "raspberry."
      3. **By 5 months**, laughing and monosyllables appear, such as "da," "ba," or
         "ga."
      4. **Between 6 and 8 months**, infants begin polysyllabic babbling, consisting
         of the same syllable repeated, such as "mamama," "dadadada."
      5. **By 9 months**, infants sporadically say "mama" or "dada" without knowing
         the meaning of these sounds.
      6. **By 10 months of age**, infants use "mama" and "dada" consistently to label
         the appropriate parent.
      7. **By 12 months**, infants acquire one or two words other than "mama," or
         "dada".
      8. **During the second year of life**, vocabulary growth velocity accelerates,
         starting at one new word per week at 12 months of age and increasing to
         one or more new words per day by 24 months of age.
      9. **By 18 to 20 months**, a toddler should be using a minimum of 20 words;
         the 24-month-old should have a vocabulary of at least 50 words.
      10. **Early during the second year of life** toddlers produce jargon, consisting
          of strings of different sounds, with rising and falling, speech-like inflection.
          These speech inflection patterns of are referred to as prosody.
      11. **By 24 months of age**, toddlers are producing two-word phrases, such as
          "want milk!"
      12. **In the second year of life**, pronouns appear ("me" and "you").
      13. **Third year.** Vocabulary growth velocity reaches a rate of several new
          words per day. A 30-month-old's vocabulary should be too large for the
          parent to count (>150 words).
      14. **By 24 to 30 months**, children develop "telegraphic" speech, which
          consists of three-to five-word sentences.
      15. **By 2 years,** the child's speech should be one-half intelligible; by 3 years,
          it should be three-fourths intelligible, and it should be completely intelligible
          by age 4 years.
   B. Auditory receptive language development
      1. **Newborn infants** respond to vocal stimuli by eye widening or changes in
         sucking rate.
      2. **The 2- or 3-month-old infant** watches and listens intently to adults and

may vocalize back.

3. **By 4 months of age** the normal infant will turn his head to locate the source of a voice; turning to inanimate stimuli, such as a bell, occurs 1 month later.
4. **By 7 to 9 months of age**, an infant will attend selectively to his own name.
5. **By 9 months of age**, infants comprehend the word "no."
6. **By 1 year of age**, infants respond to one-step commands such as "Give it to me."
7. **By 2 years of age**, toddlers can follow novel two-step commands. (eg, "Put away your shoes, then go sit down").
8. **By 2 years**, children will point to objects on command and name simple objects on command.
9. **By 36 months**, a child's receptive vocabulary includes 800 words, expanding to 1500-2000 words by age 5.
10. **By 5 years**, children are able to follow three- and four-step commands.

C. **Visual language development**
1. **During the first few weeks**, the infant will display alert visual fixation.
2. **By 4 to 6 weeks**, a social smile appears.
3. **By age 4 to 5 months**, the infant will turn towards a voice.
4. **By 6 to 7 months**, infants play gesture games, such as patty cake and peek-a-boo.
5. **Between 8 and 9 months**, infants reciprocate and eventually initiate gesture games.
6. **By 9 months**, infants appropriately wave bye-bye on command.
7. **Between 9 and 12 months**, infants express their desire for an object by reaching and crying.
8. **By 12 months**, infants indicate desired objects by pointing with the index finger.

II. **Classification of speech and language disorders**
A. **Hearing loss**
1. One infant per thousand is born with bilateral, severe-to-profound hearing loss. Two children per thousand are deafened during the first 3 years of life.
2. One third of congenital deafness is genetic in origin, one third is nongenetic, and one third is of unknown etiology. The most common nongenetic cause of deafness is fetal CMV infection.
3. Otitis media with effusion (OME) causes transient, mild-to-moderate hearing loss. Developmental language disorders (DLD) have an with increased frequency among infants with frequent OMEs.

B. **Mental retardation**
1. Three percent of children are mentally retarded, and all children who are mentally retarded are language-delayed. Mental retardation (MR) is defined as significantly subaverage general intellectual function plus delayed adaptive skills in the first 5 years of life.
2. Intelligence that is "significantly subaverage" is defined as more than 2 standard deviations (SD) below the mean. "Mild" MR is defined as -2 to -3 SD. Intelligence tests are standardized to a mean score of 100, and mild MR is equivalent to an intelligence quotient (IQ) of 69 to 55. Moderate MR = -3 to -4 SD (IQ 54 to 40), severe MR = -4 to -5 SD (IQ 39 to 25), and below -5 SD is profound MR (IQ <25).

C. **Developmental language disorders (DLD)**
1. DLD are disorders characterized by selective impairment of speech and/or language development. General intelligence is normal. DLD affects 5-10%

of preschool children, and affected boys outnumber affected girls by 3:1.

2. In the majority of cases, the etiology of DLD remains unknown; however, DLD can be caused by sex chromosome aneuploidy, fragile X syndrome, neonatal intracranial hemorrhage, fetal alcohol effects, head trauma, or human immunodeficiency virus encephalopathy. Hearing loss due to otitis media with effusion in the first 12 months of life is a possible cause of DLD.

3. **Autism.** Autism manifests as delayed and deviant language development, impaired affective development, monotonously repetitious behaviors with an insistence on routines, and an onset before 30 months of age. The prevalence is 0.2%. Autism can be caused by most of the same etiologies that cause MR.

4. **Stuttering**
   a. **Physiologic dysfluency** is characterized by a transient loss of normal rate and rhythm of speech, and it is normal in children between 2 and 4 years of age. Physiologic disfluency involves repetition of whole words ("I want . . . I want . . . I want to go home").
   b. **Stuttering** involves repetition of shorter speech segments ("I wu . . . wu . . . wwwant to go home") or a complete inability to initiate a word, referred to as "blockage." The prevalence of stuttering peaks at 4% between 2 and 4 years of age and declines to 1% among older children and adults.

5. **Dysarthria** is caused by a physical impairment of the muscles of speech production. Dysarthria in children usually is caused by cerebral palsy (CP).

III. **Clinical evaluation of speech and language disorders**
   A. **Infants with hearing-impairment.** Deaf infants coo and babble normally until 6 months of age. Thereafter, vocal output gradually diminishes.
   B. **Mentally retarded children** manifest delay in all language areas. Cooing and babbling may be reduced and delayed.
   C. **Developmental language delay** presents with expressive and receptive impairment, such as impaired intelligibility and delayed emergence of sentence structure. Speech may be effortful and reduced in amount.
   D. **Autistic children** manifest delayed and deviant language, impaired affective development, and repetitious behaviors with an insistence on routines. Autistic type language disorder is marked by impaired pragmatics--failure to use language as a medium of social interaction.
      1. Impaired social interaction may be evident from infancy, with failure to make eye contact, to engage in reciprocal vocalization, or to point to desired objects. Speech consists mainly of rhetorical naming of objects and echolalia (repetition of the utterances of others).
      2. The autistic child fails to give or receive affection.

IV. **Diagnostic evaluation of speech and language disorders**
   A. **Developmental testing** by a speech/language pathologist should be undertaken once speech or language delay has been detected.
   B. **Audiologic testing** is indicated for all children with a sign of a speech or language disorder.
   C. **Karyotype and DNA probe studies for fragile X** are indicated in children who have mental retardation, autism, or developmental language disorder.
   D. **Human immunodeficiency virus (HIV) serology** is recommended in higher risk speech-delayed children to exclude HIV encephalopathy.
   E. **Creatine kinase** measurement to exclude Duchenne muscular dystrophy is indicated for boys who have speech delay plus gross motor delay but who do not have increased deep tendon reflexes.
   F. **Cranial MRI** is indicated in the presence of focal neurologic abnormalities or

dysmorphic features suggestive of a structural brain abnormality (eg, hypertelorism, midfacial hypoplasia, aberrant hair patterning).

V. **Management of speech and language disorders.** The child who has DLD should be referred for speech therapy. Stuttering requires referral to a speech pathologist. Permanent hearing loss is treated with amplification. Therapy for autism is directed at enhancing communication and social skills.

References, see page 182.

Cardiac Disorders

Heart Murmurs

Ninety percent of children will have an audible heart murmur at some point in time. Normal murmurs include vibratory and pulmonary flow murmurs, venous hums, carotid bruits, and the murmur of physiologic branch pulmonary artery stenosis. Less than 5% of heart murmurs in children are caused by cardiac pathology.

I. **Clinical evaluation of heart murmurs**
   A. Cyanosis, exercise intolerance, feeding difficulties, dyspnea, or syncope signify potential cardiac dysfunction. Failure to thrive, diffuse diaphoresis, unexplained persistent irritability or lethargy, and atypical chest pain also suggest the possibility of organic heart disease.
   B. The majority of children who have heart murmurs are asymptomatic. In early infancy, however, cardiac malformations may manifest as persistent peaceful tachypnea (a respiratory rate greater than 60 breaths/min).

Syndromes and Associated Cardiac Malformations		
Syndrome	**Incidence of Cardiac Malformations (%)**	**Cardiac Malformations**
Down Syndrome	50	AVSD, VSD, ASD, PDA, TOF
Trisomy 18	99	VSD, PDA, DORV, BPV
Trisomy 13	90	VSD, ASD, PDA
Turner Syndrome	40	Aortic coarctation, AVS, HLH
Noonan Syndrome	50	PVS, HCM
William Syndrome	90	SVAS, SVPS, RAS
Marfan Syndrome	60-80	MVP, AoRD, AI
DiGeorge Syndrome	90	IAA (B), TA
VACTERL	80	VSD, ASD, PDA, TOF

AVSD = atrioventricular septal or canal defect, VSD = ventricular septal defect, ASD = atrial septal defect, PDA = patent ductus arteriosus, TOF = tetralogy of Fallot, DORV = double outlet right ventricle, BPV = bicuspid pulmonary valve, AVS = aortic valve stenosis, HLH = hypoplastic left heart, PVS = pulmonary valve stenosis, HCM = hypertrophic cardiomyopathy, SVAS = supravalvular aortic stenosis, SVPS = supravalvular pulmonary stenosis, RAS = renal artery stenosis, MVP = mitral valve prolapse, AoRD = aortic root dilatation, AI = aortic insufficiency, IAA (B) = interrupted

   C. **Family history** of a congenital cardiovascular malformation increases the risk of a cardiac defect, such as with DiGeorge syndrome (type B interrupted aortic arch, truncus arteriosus).
   D. **Gestational course** should be reviewed for exposure to teratogens or maternal illnesses. Fetal exposure to lithium may cause Ebstein anomaly of the tricuspid valve. Ventricular and atrial septal defects occur with fetal alcohol syndrome. Transient hypertrophic cardiomyopathy and tetralogy of Fallot are associated with maternal diabetes. Maternal collagen vascular disease may lead to fetal

complete heart block.

II. Physical examination

A. Noncardiac malformations. Twenty-five percent of children who have heart disease have extracardiac anomalies.

B. Major gastrointestinal malformations (diaphragmatic hernia, tracheoesophageal fistula and esophageal atresia, omphalocele, imperforate anus) are associated with congenital cardiac defects in 15-25% of infants. The most common cardiac malformations are ventricular septal defect and tetralogy of Fallot.

C. Cyanotic infants or children, abnormal rate or pattern of breathing, a persistently hyperdynamic precordium, precordial bulging, or asymmetric pulses should be referred to a cardiologist. Signs of congestive heart failure (inappropriate tachycardia, tachypnea, hepatomegaly, abnormal pulse volume) also should prompt referral to a cardiologist.

D. Auscultatory criteria signifying cardiac disease
   1. Loud, pansystolic, late systolic, diastolic, or continuous murmurs; an abnormally loud or single second heart sound
   2. Fourth heart sound or S_4 gallop
   3. Ejection or midsystolic clicks

Characteristics of Organic Murmurs				
Lesion	Shape	Timing	Location	Other Findings
Ventricular septal defect	Plateau	Holosystolic	LLSB	Apical mid-diastolic murmur
Mitral regurgitation	Plateau	Holosystolic	Apex	Higher pitched than VSD murmur
Atrial septal defect	Ejection	Systolic	ULSB	Persistent S2 split
Patent ductus arteriosus	Diamond	Continuous	ULSB	Bounding pulses
Aortic valve stenosis	Ejection	Systolic	URSB	Ejection click
Subvalvular aortic stenosis	Ejection	Systolic	ML-URSB	No ejection click
Hypertrophic cardiomyopathy	Ejection	Systolic	LLSB- apex	Laterally displaced PMI
Coarctation	Ejection	Systolic	ULSB-Left back	Pulse disparity
Pulmonary valve stenosis	Ejection	Systolic	ULSB	Ejection click; wide S2 split
Tetralogy of Fallot	Ejection	Systolic	MLSB	Cyanosis

Lesion	Shape	Timing	Location	Other Findings

LLSB = lower left sternal border, ULSB = upper left sternal border, URSB = upper right sternal border, MLSB = mid-left sternal border, S2 = second heart sound, PMI = point of maximal impulse.

- E. **Ventricular septal defect (VSD)** is a harsh pansystolic murmur of even amplitude that is audible at the lower left sternal border.
- F. **Patent ductus arteriosus (PDA)** causes a murmur that is continuous, louder in systole, and located at the upper left sternal border.
- G. **Ejection (crescendo-decrescendo) murmurs** are caused by ventricular outflow obstruction. Ejection murmurs begin after the first heart sound.

III. **Differentiation of normal from pathologic murmurs**
- A. **Criteria for diagnosis of a normal heart murmur**
  1. Asymptomatic patient.
  2. No evidence of associated cardiac abnormalities, extracardiac congenital malformations, or syndromes.
  3. Auscultatory features are characteristic of an innocent murmur.

Normal Murmurs					
Type	Shape	Timing	Pitch	Location	Other Findings
Vibratory	Ejection	Midsystolic	Low	LLSB-apex	Intensity ≤ grade II
Venous hum	Diamond	Continuous	Medium	Subclavicular	Disappears in supine position
Pulmonary flow	Flow	Systolic	Medium	ULSB	Normal S2 split
Physiologic branch pulmonary artery stenosis	Ejection	Systolic	Medium	Entire chest	Disappears by 4 to 6 months of age

LLSB = lower left sternal border, ULSB = upper left sternal border, S2 = second heart sound.

IV. **Heart murmurs in the newborn infant**
- A. Sixty percent of healthy term newborn infants have normal heart murmurs. One third of neonates who have serious heart malformations may not have a detectable heart murmur during the first 2 weeks of life. Thirty percent of newborn infants subsequently determined to have heart disease are discharged from the newborn nursery as ostensibly healthy.
- B. **Persistent peaceful tachypnea** should not be dismissed; 90% of infants who have serious cardiac disease have persistent tachypnea after birth.
- C. **A persistently hyperdynamic precordium** suggests organic heart disease.
- D. **Auscultation of the second heart sound.** In healthy neonates, the second heart sound is split audibly by 12 hours of age. A single second heart sound in

a quiet neonate indicates: 1) the absence of one outflow tract valve (aortic or pulmonary atresia); 2) an abnormal position of the great vessels (transposition of the great arteries or tetralogy of Fallot); or 3) pulmonary hypertension (ventricular defect, persistent pulmonary hypertension).

References, see page 182.

Chest Pain in Children

Chest pain is the presenting complaint in 6 per 1,000 children who present to pediatric emergency departments or walk-in clinics. Young children are more likely to have a cardiorespiratory cause of their pain, such as cough, asthma, pneumonia, or heart disease; adolescents are more likely to have pain associated with a psychogenic disturbance.

I. **Differential diagnosis of chest pain in children**
   A. **Cardiac disease**
      1. Cardiac disease is a rare cause of chest pain in children. However, myocardial infarction can rarely result from anomalous coronary arteries. Some children will have a pansystolic, continuous, or mitral regurgitation murmur or gallop rhythm that suggests myocardial dysfunction.
      2. Arrhythmias may cause palpitations or abnormalities on cardiac examination. Supraventricular tachycardia is the most common arrhythmia, but premature ventricular beats or tachycardia also can cause episodes of brief sharp chest pain.
      3. **Hypertrophic obstructive cardiomyopathy** is an autosomal dominant structural disorder; therefore, there often is a family history of the condition. Children may have a murmur that may be audible when standing or when performing a Valsalva maneuver. These patients are at risk for ischemic chest pain.
      4. **Mitral valve prolapse** may cause chest pain secondary to papillary muscle or endocardial ischemia. A midsystolic click and a late systolic murmur may be detected.
      5. **Cardiac infections** are uncommon causes of pediatric chest pain.
         a. **Pericarditis** presents with sharp, stabbing pain that improves when the patient sits up and leans forward. The child usually is febrile; is in respiratory distress; and has a friction rub, distant heart sounds, neck vein distention, and pulsus paradoxus.
         b. **Myocarditis** presents as mild pain that has been present for several days. After a few days of fever, vomiting and lightheadedness, the patient may develop pain or shortness of breath on exertion. Examination may reveal muffled heart sounds, fever, a gallop rhythm, or tachycardia. The patient also may have orthostatic changes in pulse or blood pressure.
         c. **Chest radiography** will show cardiomegaly in both of these infections, and the electrocardiogram will be abnormal. An echocardiogram will confirm the diagnosis.

Cardiac Disorders Leading to Pediatric Chest Pain
Coronary Artery Disease--Ischemia/Infarction
<ul><li>Anomalous coronary arteries</li><li>Coronary arteritis (Kawasaki disease)</li><li>Long-standing diabetes mellitus</li></ul>
Arrhythmia
<ul><li>Supraventricular tachycardia</li><li>Ventricular tachycardia</li></ul>
Structural Abnormalities
<ul><li>Hypertrophic cardiomyopathy</li><li>Severe pulmonic stenosis</li><li>Aortic valve stenosis</li><li>Mitral valve prolapse</li></ul>
Infection
<ul><li>Pericarditis</li><li>Myocarditis</li></ul>

- B. **Musculoskeletal pain**
    1. Musculoskeletal pain is one of the most common diagnoses in children who have chest discomfort. Children frequently strain chest wall muscles while exercising.
    2. **Trauma** to the chest may result in a mild contusion or a rib fracture. The physical examination will reveal chest tenderness.
    3. **Costochondritis** is common in children, and it is characterized by tenderness over the costochondral junctions. The pain is sharp and exaggerated by physical activity or breathing.
- C. **Respiratory conditions**
    1. **Severe cough, asthma, or pneumonia** may cause chest pain because of overuse of chest wall muscles. Crackles, wheezes, tachypnea, or decreased breath sounds are present.
    2. **Exercise-induced asthma** may cause chest pain, which can be confirmed with a treadmill test.
    3. **Spontaneous pneumothorax or pneumomediastinum** may occasionally cause chest pain with respiratory distress. Children with asthma, cystic fibrosis or Marfan syndrome are at high risk for these conditions. Signs include respiratory distress, decreased breath sounds on the affected side, and palpable subcutaneous air.
    4. **Pulmonary embolism** is extremely rare in pediatric patients, but it should be considered in the adolescent girl who has dyspnea, fever, pleuritic pain, cough, and hemoptysis. Oral contraceptives or recent abortion increase the risk. Young males who have had recent leg trauma also are at risk.
- D. **Psychogenic chest pain** may present with hyperventilation or an anxious appearance. A recent stressful event (separation from friends, parental

divorce, school failure) may often be related temporally to the onset of the chest pain.

E. **Gastrointestinal disorders**
1. **Reflux esophagitis** often causes chest pain which is described as burning, substernal, and worsened by reclining or eating spicy foods. This condition is confirmed with a therapeutic trial of antacids.
2. **Foreign body ingestion** may cause chest pain when the object lodges in the esophagus. A radiograph confirms the diagnosis.

F. **Miscellaneous causes of pediatric chest pain**
1. **Sickle cell disease** may cause an acute chest syndrome.
2. **Marfan syndrome** may cause chest pain and fatal abdominal aortic aneurysm dissection.
3. **Collagen vascular disorders** may cause chest pain and pleural effusions.
4. **Shingles** may cause chest pain that precedes or occurs simultaneously with the rash.
5. **Coxsackievirus infection** may lead to pleurodynia with paroxysms of sharp chest pain.
6. **Breast tenderness during puberty or early breast changes of pregnancy** may present as chest pain.
7. **Idiopathic chest pain.** No diagnosis can be determined in 20-45% of cases of pediatric chest pain.

II. **Clinical evaluation of chest pain**
A. **A history and physical examination** will reveal the etiology of chest pain in most cases. The history may reveal asthma, previous heart disease, or Kawasaki disease. Family history may reveal familial hypertrophic obstructive cardiomyopathy.
B. **The frequency and severity of the pain** and whether the pain interrupts the child's daily activity should be determined. Pain that wakes the child from sleep is more likely to be related to an organic etiology.
C. **Burning pain** in the sternal area suggests esophagitis. Sharp stabbing pain that is relieved by sitting up and leaning forward suggests pericarditis in a febrile child.
D. **Mode of onset of pain.** Acute onset of pain is more likely to represent an organic etiology. Chronic pain is much more likely to have a idiopathic or psychogenic origin.
E. **Precipitating factors**
1. **Trauma, muscle strain, or choking on a foreign body** should be sought.
2. **Exercise-induced chest pain** may be caused by cardiac disease or exercise-induced asthma.
3. **Syncope, fever or palpitations** associated with chest pain are signs of an organic etiology.
4. **Joint pain, rash, or fever** may be suggested by the presence of collagen vascular disease.
5. **Stressful conditions** at home or school should be sought.
6. **Substance abuse (cocaine) or oral contraceptives** should be sought in adolescents.
F. **Physical examination**
1. **Severe distress** warrants immediate treatment for life-threatening conditions, such as pneumothorax.
2. **Hyperventilation** may be distinguished from respiratory distress by the absence of cyanosis or nasal flaring.
3. **Pallor or poor growth** may suggest a malignancy or collagen vascular disease.

4. **Abdominal tenderness** may suggest abdominal pain that is referred to the chest.
5. **Rales, wheezes, decreased breath sounds, murmurs, rubs, muffled heart sounds, or arrhythmias** suggest a cardiopulmonary pathology.
6. **The chest wall** should be evaluated for bruises (trauma), tenderness (musculoskeletal pain), or subcutaneous air (pneumothorax or pneumomediastinum).

III. **Laboratory evaluation**
   A. **A chest radiograph** is warranted if the patient has fever, respiratory distress, or abnormal breath sounds. Fever and cardiomegaly suggests pericarditis or myocarditis.
   B. **Electrocardiography** is recommended if the pain was acute in onset (began in the last 2-3 days) or if there is an abnormal cardiac examination (unexplained tachycardia, arrhythmia, murmur, rub, or click).
   C. **Exercise stress testing or pulmonary function testing** is appropriate for evaluation of cardiac disease or asthma.
   D. **Holter monitoring** is warranted for syncope or palpitations.
   E. **Children with chronic pain**, a normal physical examination, and no history suggestive of cardiac or pulmonary disease do not require laboratory studies.
   F. **Blood counts and sedimentation rates** are of value if collagen vascular disease, infection, or malignancy is suspected.
   G. **Drug screening** may be indicated in the older child who has acute pain associated with anxiety, tachycardia, hypertension, or shortness of breath.

IV. **Management of pediatric chest pain**
   A. **Emergency department referral** is necessary if the child is in severe distress or has a history of significant trauma.
   B. **Referral to a cardiologist** is recommended for children with known or suspected heart disease, syncope, palpitations, or pain on exertion.
   C. **Musculoskeletal, psychogenic, or idiopathic pain** usually will respond to reassurance, analgesics, rest, and application of a heating pad. If esophagitis is suspected, a trial of antacids may be beneficial.

References, see page 182.

Allergic and Dermatologic Disorders

Asthma

Asthma is a chronic lung disease caused by inflammation and bronchospasm. The disorder manifests as recurrent cough, wheezing, shortness of breath, reduced expiratory flow, exercise intolerance, and respiratory distress. Asthma affects 4-5% of children. Symptoms usually begin in the first 5 years of life, and many children improve during adolescence.

I. **Pathogenesis**
   A. Treatment of asthma is aimed at preventing and minimizing inflammation. Airway inflammation is caused by allergy, infection, and irritants. Inflammation causes increased mucus, swollen, thickened bronchioles, and bronchospasm.
   B. Most children have only occasional symptoms; a few children are constantly symptomatic.

II. **Prevention of acute asthma**
   A. **Influenza** can trigger asthma symptoms; therefore, asthmatic children should receive influenza vaccine annually.
   B. **Cigarette smoke** is a significant trigger of asthma, and nicotine nasal spray may help patients and parents stop smoking.
   C. **Allergens** may trigger asthma. Air filters and air conditioning are helpful.
   D. **Allergens.** Seasonal allergic asthma is often provoked by ragweed, grasses, and pollen. Perennial asthma is often provoked by molds, goose down, feathers, dust, and cat and dog dander. Furry pets should be kept outdoors.
   E. **Microscopic dust mites** may trigger asthma. Measures that reduce exposure include removal of carpet and stuffed animals, replacement of feather pillows with Dacron, laundering bedding weekly, encasing mattress and pillows in vinyl, vacuuming and damp dusting, and use of an acaricide.
   F. **Exercise**, especially in cold, dry air, triggers symptoms in 90% of asthmatics. Symptoms can be reduced by warming up, breathing through the nose, and covering the nose and mouth with a scarf when exercising in the cold.
   G. **Infections.** Colds and sinus infections are common asthma triggers.

III. **Treatment of chronic asthma symptoms**
   A. Treatment for asthma focuses on anti-inflammatory medications such as cromolyn, nedocromil, and steroids. Beta-agonists are second-line treatment, which are used to control symptom flare-ups.
   B. For older children, metered dose inhalers (MDIs) are the best way to administer medications, but they are effective only if used as follows:
      1. Shake canister while taking a deep breath in and out.
      2. Hold can 1 inch from mouth.
      3. Depress button at the beginning of the next inhalation.
      4. Breathe the mist in deeply and hold breath to count of 10; exhale.
   C. Children should be provided a spacer. Nebulized solutions are needed only for children who are too young to use MDIs.

IV. **Medications**
   A. **Mast cell stabilizers**
      1. Inhaled cromolyn and nedocromil are mast cell stabilizers that inhibit histamine release. These agents are the mainstays of chronic asthma management. Cromolyn and nedocromil must be taken consistently to be effective; they are not effective in acute attacks.

2. **Cromolyn (Intal)** is given as 2 puffs, four times daily. After resolution of symptoms, the frequency may be reduced to tid. It is available in nebulizer solution, aerosol or MDI, and spinhaler.

3. **Nedocromil (Tilade)** is approved for children 12 years and older. Treatment begins with 2 puffs, qid and may be reduced to tid or bid.

B. **Inhaled steroids**

1. Inhaled steroids are effective for prevention and treatment of moderate or severe asthma in children 6 years of age and older. If given when peak flow meter readings start to fall, steroids can prevent exacerbations. Inhaled steroids do not affect growth. They can cause throat irritation and hoarseness. Side effects can be reduced by using a spacer and by gargling with water after administration.

2. **Beclomethasone (Beclovent)** is administered as 2-4 puffs bid.

3. **Triamcinolone (Azmacort)** is given as 2-4 puffs bid.

4. **Flunisolide (AeroBid)** is given as 2-4 puffs bid.

5. A low-strength steroid (beclomethasone) should be used first, and a more potent preparation (triamcinolone, flunisolide) should be used if symptoms continue.

C. **Beta-agonists**

1. The beta-agonists (eg, albuterol [Ventolin, Proventil]) are effective bronchodilators, reducing symptoms within 30 minutes when given by aerosol. They are useful for the rapid relief of exacerbations. Beta-agonist medications are used to supplement anti-inflammatory medications and to prevent flare-ups.

2. Oral administration is significantly less effective than inhaled treatments, and there are more systemic side effects, including anorexia, hypertension, tachycardia, and jitteriness.

3. **Salmeterol (Serevent)**, a longer-acting (12-hour) beta-agonist medication, is more effective than albuterol, but it has been approved only for use by teenagers and adults. Salmeterol has a long half-life, and it should not be used as a "rescue" medication. Salmeterol is indicated for teenagers who have moderate or severe asthma, require a relatively constant daily dose of beta-agonist, and can take it regularly every 12 hours.

Dosages of Drugs for Acute Severe Exacerbation of Asthma		
Medications	**Dosages**	**Comments**
Sympathomimetics Metered dose inhaler 90 mcg/puff	6-10 puffs every 20 min for three doses, then every 1-4 h as needed	Nebulization is preferred for patients in severe distress
Albuterol Nebulizer solution (5 mg/mL)	0.15 mg/kg (minimum dose, 2.5 mg) every 20 min for 3 doses, then 0.15-0.3 mg/kg or 2.5-10 mg every 1-4 h as needed	Dilute to minimum of 4 mL and maximum of 6 mL; flow at 6-12 L/min

Corticosteroids Prednisone Methylprednisolone	1 mg/kg every 6 h for 48 h, then 1-2 mg/kg/day in 2 divided doses until PEF is 70% of predicted normal or personal best	For outpatient "burst," use 1-2 mg/kg/day with a maximum of 60 mg for 3-7 days

  D. Oral steroids
   1. Oral corticosteroids may be required for severe asthma. Side effects include decreased growth, unstable blood glucose levels, impaired immunity, and adrenocortical suppression.
   2. Steroids should be administered for as short a time as possible (eg, 3-5 days for acute symptoms). The dose should be given in the morning when endogenous corticosteroid levels are highest. The frequency should be reduced to every other day as soon as possible.
   3. Children on continuous steroid therapy who develop varicella should be given acyclovir to reduce the risk of severe disease.
  E. Theophylline and aminophylline
   1. Theophylline and aminophylline have some anti-inflammatory and bronchodilator activity. Side effects include hyperactivity, decreased attention span, decreased appetite, and increased risk of seizures.
   2. Theophylline is useful in only two settings: 1) children younger than 6 years who have chronic asthma and whose parents are unable to manage frequent nebulizer treatments, 2) children of any age who have moderate-to-severe asthma and who are already are taking cromolyn or nedocromil, inhaled steroids, and a beta-agonist, but who remain symptomatic and for whom the only other alternative is daily systemic corticosteroid medication.
V. Peak flow monitoring
  A. Daily home peak flow meter readings should be maintained in the green zone (>80% of predicted peak flow). Yellow zone results (50-79%) indicate the need to augment baseline therapy. Peak flows in the red zone indicate the need for urgent medical evaluation and treatment.

References, see page 182.

Contact Dermatitis

Contact dermatitis is an extremely common occurrence in the pediatric age group. There are two major forms of contact dermatitis: irritant and allergic. Irritant contact dermatitis is the most common and occurs when a person is exposed to an agent that has a direct toxic effect on the skin. Common causes of irritant contact dermatitis include overbathing, drooling, prolonged contact with moisture and feces in the diaper, and bubble baths.

I. Clinical evaluation
   A. Contact dermatitis usually first appears in infants 2-6 months of age. Infants and children have rashes on the shoulders, chest, abdomen, and back. Infants usually also have a rash on the face, scalp and around the ears. Children older than 18 months old tend to have rashes on the neck and antecubital and popliteal fossae. Contact dermatitis usually resolves by puberty, but it sometimes recurs at times of stress.
   B. Acute lesions are itchy, red, edematous papules and small vesicles which may progress to weeping and crusting lesions. Chronic rubbing and scratching may cause lichenification and hyperpigmentation. The classic triad of atopy consists of asthma, allergic rhinitis, and dermatitis.

Precipitating Factors and Activities in Contact Dermatitis	
Moisture-related	Excessive bathing, excessive hand washing, excessive lip licking, excessive sweating, extended showers or baths, repeated contact with water, swimming, occlusive clothing and footwear
Contact-related	Overuse of soap, bubble-bath, cosmetics, deodorants, detergents, solvents, tight clothing, rough fabrics, wool or mohair
Temperature-related	Exposure to excessive warmth, humidity, overdressing, hot showers or baths
Emotional	Anger, anxiety, depression, stress
Infective	Bacteria, fungi, viruses
Inhalational	Animal dander, cigarette smoke, dust, perfume

   C. Patch testing is useful for evaluation of persistent, localized reactions of the hands, feet, and perioral area. It also may be useful in patients who have atopic dermatitis and experience a flare or persistence of disease despite appropriate therapy.

II. Treatment of contact dermatitis
   A. Moisture. Avoidance of excessive bathing, hand washing, and lip licking is recommended. Showers or baths should be limited to no more than 5 minutes. After bathing, patients should apply a moisturizer (Aquaphor, Eucerin, Lubriderm,

petrolatum) to noninflamed skin.

B. Contact with irritants

1. Overuse of soap should be discouraged. Use of nonirritating soaps (eg, Dove, Ivory, Neutrogena) should be limited to the axilla, groin, hands, and feet.
2. Infants often have bright red exudative contact dermatitis (slobber dermatitis) on the cheeks, resulting from drooling. A corticosteroid will usually bring improvement.

C. Topical corticosteroids

1. Corticosteroid ointments maintain skin hydration and maximize penetration. Corticosteroid creams may sting when applied to acute lesions.
2. Mid- and low-potency topical corticosteroids are used twice-daily for chronic, atopic dermatitis. High-potency steroids may be used for flare-ups, but the potency should be tapered after the dermatitis is controlled.
3. Use of high-potency agents on the face, genitalia and skin-folds may cause epidermal atrophy ("stretch marks"), rebound erythema, and susceptibility to bruising.

Commonly Used Topical Corticosteroids	
Preparation	**Size**
Low-Potency Agents	
Hydrocortisone ointment, cream, 1, 2.5% (Hytone)	30 g
Mild-Potency Agents	
Alclometasone dipropionate cream, ointment, 0.05% (Aclovate)	60 g
Triamcinolone acetonide cream, 0.1% (Aristocort)	60 g
Fluocinolone acetonide cream, 0.01% (Synalar)	60 g
Medium-Potency Agents	
Triamcinolone acetonide ointment (Aristocort A), 0.1%	60 g
Betamethasone dipropionate cream (Diprosone), 0.05%	45 g
Triamcinolone acetonide cream, ointment, 0.1% (Kenalog)	60 g
Mometasone cream 0.1% (Elocon)	45 g
Fluocinolone acetonide ointment, 0.025% (Synalar)	60 g
Hydrocortisone butyrate 0.1% cream, ointment (Locoid)	45 g
Betamethasone valerate cream, 0.1% (Valisone)	45 g
Hydrocortisone valerate cream, ointment, 0.2% (Westcort)	60 g

Preparation	Size
High-Potency Agents	
Amcinonide ointment, 0.1% (Cyclocort)	60 g
Betamethasone dipropionate ointment (Diprosone) 0.05%	45 g
Fluocinonide cream, ointment, 0.05% (Lidex)	60 g

4. **Allergic reactions to topical corticosteroids** may occur. Mometasone (Elocon) is the least likely to cause an allergic reaction.
D. **Antihistamines**, such as diphenhydramine or hydroxyzine (Atarax), are somewhat useful for pruritus and are sedating. Nonsedating antihistamines, such as loratadine (Claritin) and fexofenadine (Allegra), are helpful.
E. **Systemic steroids.** Systemic corticosteroids are reserved for severe, widespread reactions to poison ivy, or for severe involvement of the hands, face, or genitals. Prednisone, 1-2 mg/kg, is given PO and tapered over 10-18 days.

References, see page 182.

Diaper Dermatitis

Diaper rash is one of the most common skin disorders, occurring in 50% of infants, with 5% having severe rash. The peak incidence is between 9 and 12 months of age.

I. **Pathophysiology**. Breast fed infants have fewer diaper rashes than formula-fed infants. The frequency and severity of diaper dermatitis are significantly lower when the number of diaper changes per day is eight or more. Superabsorbent disposable diapers significantly reduce the severity of diaper rash when compared to cloth diapers.
II. **Classification of diaper dermatitis**
   A. **Dermatoses related to diaper wearing**
      1. **Irritant diaper dermatitis** is the most common form of diaper dermatitis. It is accentuated on the convex areas, including the buttocks, lower abdomen, genitalia, and upper thigh, sparing the creases. It varies in severity from mild erythema (with or without scales) to papules and macerated lesions.
         a. **Management**
            (1) Irritant diaper dermatitis can best be prevented by keeping the skin in the diaper area protected from urine and feces by increasing the frequency of diaper changes and by using superabsorbent disposable diapers.
            (2) A low-potency corticosteroid ointment (hydrocortisone 1%) should be applied four times daily with diaper changes. Anticandidal agents such as nystatin (Mycostatin), clotrimazole (Lotrimin), or ketoconazole (Nizoral) should also be added.
            (3) Thickly applied barrier creams, such as A&D ointment, zinc oxide pastes or Vaseline, may be helpful.

2. **Candidal diaper dermatitis**
   a. Candidal diaper dermatitis is characterized by beefy red plaques with white scales and satellite papules and pustules, which almost always involve the inguinal creases. It often develops after an episode of diarrhea or after use of antibiotics. KOH scrapings may demonstrate pseudohyphae.
   b. Candidiasis is treated with topical nystatin (Mycostatin), clotrimazole (Lotrimin), miconazole (Monistat), or ketoconazole (Nizoral) applied 3-4 times daily. Hydrocortisone 1% ointment may help decrease erythema and inflammation and can be applied at the same time. Oral nystatin (Mycostatin) suspension, four times a day, should be used if repeated episodes of candidal dermatitis occur. The mother should be evaluated for candidal infection of the nipples or genital tract. In severe cases, oral fluconazole 3 mg/kg per day as a pulse dose weekly x 2 or for a short course of 5 to 7 days may be of benefit.

References, see page 182.

Dermatophyte Infections

Dermatophytes constitute a group of about 40 fungal species that cause superficial infections called dermatophytoses, ringworm, or tinea.

I. **Tinea capitis**
   A. Tinea capitis presents as inflammation with hair breakage and loss. Inflammatory changes can range from minimal scaling and redness that resembles mild seborrhea to tenderness, redness, edema, purulence, and hair loss (kerion).
   B. A hypersensitivity reaction to fungal antigen can develop, called a dermatophytid or "id" reaction. Id reactions can present with either a dermatitis that includes redness, superficial edema involving the epidermis, and scaling or with a "pityriasis rosea-like" reaction that involves red, scaly papules and ovoid plaques on the face, neck, trunk, and proximal extremities.
   C. Topical antifungals are not effective for hair infection. Griseofulvin is preferred for initial treatment at a starting dose of about 20 mg/kg per day.
   D. Selenium sulfide shampoo (Selsun Blue) is used in conjunction with oral antifungals to reduce contagion. Tinea capitis is contagious until after 2 weeks of systemic treatment. Dermatophytid reactions can be treated with topical corticosteroids.
II. **Tinea corporis (ring worm) and tinea cruris**
   A. Dermatophyte infection of the body surface is termed tinea corporis. Tinea cruris describes infection of the upper thigh and inguinal area. Examination reveals red, scaly papules and small plaques. These progressively enlarge to form expanding rings, arcs, or annular patterns.
   B. Clearing in previously affected areas produces the typical "ringworm" appearance. Topical therapy is the initial treatment approach.
III. **Tinea pedis and tinea manuum**
   A. Tinea pedis infection is often interdigital and is induced by the warmth and moisture of wearing shoes. The web spaces become red and scaly. Fungal infection frequently spreads to involve the soles of the feet or the palms, with dry scale and minimal redness. Scaling extends to the side of the foot or hand. Vesicle and blister formation and itching are common.

B. Dermatophyte infection often leads to secondary bacterial infection. A dermatophytid reaction may occur, as described for tinea capitis.

C. Dermatophyte hand infection presents as dry scale on the palm. Infection of just one hand in conjunction with infection of both feet is the most common pattern.

D. Topical therapy and keeping the involved areas as dry as possible is recommended for hand or foot tinea. Oral therapy may be necessary for recalcitrant disease.

IV. Onychomycosis (tinea unguium)

A. Dermatophyte infection of the nail plate is referred to as onychomycosis, characterized by dystrophy of the nail, discoloration, ridging, thickening, fragility, breakage, accumulation of debris beneath the distal aspect of the nail and little or no inflammation.

B. Oral treatment usually is required to clear infection, but recurrence is very common.

V. Diagnosis

A. **Potassium hydroxide (KOH) examination** of scale, hair, or nail is the most rapid diagnostic method. A sample of scale, hair, or nail from a possibly infected area is placed on a glass slide, covered with a few drops of 30% KOH, and gently heated. The specimen is examined for spores and/or fungal hyphae.

B. **Fungal culture** of scale and affected hair or nail can be accomplished by incubation at room temperature for 2 to 3 weeks.

VI. Treatment

A. **Oral griseofulvin** is effective and safe for treatment of tinea capitis in children. However, its erratic oral absorption necessitates doses of about 20 mg/kg per day of the liquid preparation, always administered with a fatty meal or beverage (such as milk). Ultramicrosize griseofulvin can be administered at the lower dose of 8 to 10 mg/kg per day.

B. Treatment should be continued for 8 to 12 weeks. There is no need for liver function testing when griseofulvin is used for 6 months or less. Adverse effects associated with griseofulvin include headaches and gastrointestinal upset.

Systemic Antifungal Agents
Griseofulvin 20 mg/kg per day of microsize liquid or 7 to 10 mg/kg per day of ultramicrosize tablets
Itraconazole (Sporanox) 4 to 6 mg/kg per day
Terbinafine (Lamisil) 3 to 5 mg/kg per day

Topical Treatments for Tinea Pedis, Tinea Cruris and Tinea Corporis						
Antifungal agent	**Prescription**	**Cream**	**Solution or spray**	**Lotion**	**Powder**	**Frequency of application**
Imidazoles						
Clotrimazole 1 percent (Lotrimin, Mycelex)		X	X	X		Twice daily
Miconazole 2 percent (Micatin, Monistat-Derm)		X	X	X	X	Twice daily
Econazole 1 percent (Spectazole)	X	X				Once daily
Ketoconazole 2 percent (Nizoral)	X	X	X			Once daily
Oxiconazole 1 percent (Oxistat)	X	X		X		Once daily or twice daily
Allylamines						
Naftifine 1 percent (Naftin)	X	X				Once daily or twice daily
Terbinafine 1 percent (Lamisil)	X	X	X			Once daily or twice daily
Butenafine 1 percent (Mentax)		X				Once daily or twice daily

C. **Itraconazole (Sporanox)** is effective and can be given orally at 3 to 5 mg/kg per day for 4 to 6 weeks or until clearing, followed by a 4-week period off of therapy. A liquid formulation is available.

D. **Terbinafine (Lamisil)** orally at 3 to 6 mg/kg per day for 4 to 6 weeks is effective.

E. **Topical antifungals** can be used once to twice daily to clear infections other than tinea capitis and onychomycosis. Newer, more potent topical agents with once-daily dosing can improve compliance.

F. **Hydrocortisone** 1% or 2.5% can be added to antifungal therapy to reduce inflammation. Affected areas should be kept as cool and as dry as possible.

References, see page 182.

Herpes Simplex Virus Infections

HSV is a member of the herpesvirus family, which includes varicella zoster virus, Epstein-Barr virus, and cytomegalovirus. Like all herpesviruses, HSV tends to establish latent infection and eventually it reactivates and becomes infectious. Most HSV-infected patients have asymptomatic infections or the symptoms are only mildly uncomfortable. However, a substantial number of patients experience frequent painful recurrences or severe or life-threatening illnesses.

I. **Virology and pathogenesis**
    A. Two types of HSV exist: HSV-1 and HSV-2. Both types can infect any anatomic site.
    B. **HSV-1** may cause asymptomatic infection, oral lesions, nonoral or non-genital skin lesions, encephalitis, neonatal disease, and genital lesions
    C. **HSV-2** may cause asymptomatic infection, genital lesions, neonatal disease, nonoral, nongenital skin lesions, meningitis, and oral lesions
    D. During epithelial cell infection, HSV infects the regional sensory or autonomic nerves, traveling via the nerve axon to the neuron, where it establishes a latent infection. The virus may reactivate at a later time. Factors that may cause reactivation include immunodeficiency, physical and psychosocial stress, trauma, and exposure to ultraviolet light.
    E. Seroprevalence is more common among patients in lower socioeconomic class (50-60%) than among those of middle (35%) or higher socioeconomic class (10-20%). HSV-2 infection risk among individuals reporting one sexual partner is less than 10%. Among individuals reporting 2 to 10 partners the risk is 40%.

II. **Transmission**
    A. HSV-1 and HSV-2 are transmitted from person to person through contact with infected skin lesions, mucous membranes, and secretions. The incubation period is 1 to 26 days, and both types may be transmitted in utero or perinatally.
    B. Asymptomatic virus shedding may transmit the disease. Women who have had previous genital HSV-2 infection shed virus on 2% of days.

Characteristics of Primary and Recurrent Genital HSV Infection	
Primary Infection	**Recurrent Infection**
Extensive skin lesions	Localized skin lesions
Tender inguinal adenopathy	No adenopathy
Fever, headache, other systemic symptoms	No systemic symptoms
Extragenital skin lesions	No extragenital lesions
Meningitis	Meningitis is rare
Typically, recurrence within 1 year	Recurrence within 1 year less likely

C. **Oral/facial HSV infections**
    1. HSV-1 infection is extremely common in infants and children. The most common clinical manifestation of primary HSV-1 infection is gingivostomatitis, characterized by fever, malaise, myalgia, pharyngitis, irritability, and cervical adenopathy. The illness is self-limited and usually of short duration.
    2. Recurrent HSV-1 infections are most frequently characterized by oral and lip lesions. Many individuals who have oral HSV lesions have no known

history of prior gingivostomatitis.

3. HSV-2 also may cause oral lesions and pharyngitis, particularly in sexually active individuals.

D. Genital HSV infections

1. Many HSV infections are asymptomatic, but they can also cause papular, vesicular, or ulcerative lesions with pain, itching, urethral or vaginal discharge, and dysuria.

2. Primary infections cause more severe symptoms and signs, including extensive skin lesions, tender inguinal adenopathy, and extragenital lesions. Primary infections are often associated with fever, headache, malaise, abdominal pain, and aseptic meningitis.

3. Eighty percent of persons who have a first episode of HSV-2 genital infection will experience a recurrence in the first year. Thereafter, most patients who have genital HSV infection have few symptomatic recurrences.

E. HSV encephalitis

1. HSV encephalitis is the most common viral infection of the CNS. The incidence peaks at 5 to 30 years and at more than 50 years. Ninety five percent of cases are caused by HSV-1. HSV encephalitis is characterized by acute fever, altered mental status, and focal neurologic symptoms and signs.

2. Routine CSF findings are not diagnostic. Polymerase chain reaction (PCR) can detect HSV DNA in CSF. HSV is rarely isolated by culture of the CSF.

3. Electroencephalographic (EEG) findings can be diagnostic, with spike and slow wave activity localized to the temporal region.

4. CT scan and MRI may reveal localized edema and hemorrhage suggestive of HSV infection; however, these findings occur late in the course of the illness.

5. The prognosis for HSV encephalitis without treatment is poor, and even with antiviral therapy, substantial morbidity and mortality occurs. Prompt institution of empiric therapy is essential when the clinical diagnosis is suspected.

F. Neonatal HSV infections

1. Infection in neonates results from vertical transmission during the peripartum period in 85%; *in utero* or postpartum transmission rarely occurs. Seventy percent of untreated infants will progress to disseminated or CNS disease. Most neonatal infections are caused by HSV-2, although 30% of cases are caused by HSV-1. Seventy to 80% of infected infants are born to mothers who are unaware that they have genital HSV infection.

2. **Skin, eye, mouth (SEM) disease** accounts for 45% of peripartum infections.

   a. SEM disease most commonly presents in the first or second weeks of life with vesicular skin lesions which may occur anywhere on the body. Skin lesions have an erythematous base with clear or cloudy fluid, or may appear pustular.

   b. If the infection does not progress to involve the CNS or viscera, SEM disease has a low mortality; however, recurrences occur in 90%.

3. **Central nervous system disease** is manifest as encephalitis, and it accounts for 35% of peripartum infections.

   a. Neonatal HSV CNS disease most commonly presents in the second to third week of life. Only 60% will develop skin lesions during the illness. HSV CNS disease has a 50% mortality if not treated; with treatment, mortality is 18%. The diagnosis must be considered in any infant who presents with encephalitis, seizures, apnea, bradycardia, or cranial nerve abnormalities.

    b. Cerebrospinal fluid findings are nonspecific and include pleocytosis and increased protein. Early initiation of therapy is critical when the diagnosis is suspected.

  4. Disseminated disease is characterized by hepatitis, pneumonitis, and disseminated intravascular coagulation, and it accounts for 20% of peripartum infections.

    a. HSV disseminated disease presents in the first week of life. Bilateral patchy infiltrates are indicative of pneumonitis. Skin lesions may not be present initially.

    b. Disseminated HSV disease should be considered in any infant presenting with sepsis that is unresponsive to antibiotic therapy, or who has both pneumonitis and hepatitis. Without treatment, disseminated HSV infection has an 80% mortality rate. With treatment, the mortality is reduced only to 50-60%. Pneumonitis has an 80% mortality rate with treatment.

  5. Eye infections

    a. HSV is the most common cause of corneal blindness. HSV keratitis is characterized by conjunctivitis and dendritic lesions of the cornea.

    b. Topical steroids are contraindicated because they may facilitate spread of infection to the deep structures of the eyes.

III. Management of perinatal HSV infection

  A. The most reliable predictor of the risk of perinatal transmission is whether a woman has active genital lesions at the time of delivery.

  B. A thorough physical examination, including vaginal speculum exam, at the onset of labor should exclude the presence of active genital lesions. If HSV lesions are found during labor, prompt cesarean section is recommended.

  C. Management of infants exposed to HSV at delivery

    1. Virus cultures of the infant's conjunctivae, pharynx, skin folds, CSF, and rectum at 24-48 hours can indicate whether HSV has been transmitted. Infants who are culture positive for HSV from any site after 24 hours of life are given antiretroviral therapy with acyclovir.

    2. During the time when HSV-exposed infants are in the hospital, they should be placed in contact isolation. Circumcision is deferred.

IV. Diagnosis of HSV infection

  A. HSV-1 and HSV-2 can be isolated by virus culture from active skin, eye, and genital lesions. In cases of recurrent disease, virus shedding may be too brief to be detected by virus culture. Herpes simplex is rarely is recovered from CSF by culture.

  B. Although less sensitive and specific than culture, staining for virus antigens with fluorescent antibodies detects HSV more rapidly.

  C. PCR is a useful diagnostic procedure for HSV encephalitis, with a sensitivity of 75% and a specificity of 100%.

V. Therapy for HSV infections

  A. Acyclovir is the treatment of choice for most cases of serious HSV infection and for prophylaxis. Acyclovir interferes with viral DNA polymerase.

  B. Parenteral acyclovir is indicated for severe or potentially severe infections, such as neonatal HSV infection, HSV encephalitis, and non-localized infections in immunocompromised patients. Oral acyclovir decreases new lesion formation and improves symptoms in first episode genital HSV. Oral acyclovir has limited effect on the resolution of recurrent HSV disease.

  C. Topical acyclovir is not effective for skin or oral lesions. The ophthalmic

solution is useful for HSV keratitis, in combination with IV acyclovir.
- **D. Acyclovir (Zovirax)**
    1. For serious infections, such as neonatal disease and encephalitis, 5-10 mg/kg IV is given q8h for 10 to 21 days. Doses up to 20 mg/kg IV q8h are used for infants who have CNS or disseminated infection.
    2. Oral acyclovir dosage is 20 mg/kg every 8 hours or 200 mg five times a day for 7-10 days. The adult regimen can be simplified to 400 mg three times a day.
    3. Suppression is indicated for immunocompromised patients or patients who have more than 6 genital recurrences a year; 5 mg/kg q8h or 400 mg bid. Suppressive therapy is also used for infants who have HSV SEM disease.
    4. Acyclovir is well tolerated. The most common adverse effect is gastrointestinal upset. Nephrotoxicity can be avoided by keeping the patient well hydrated.
- **E. Valacyclovir (Valtrex)** is an ester of acyclovir that has better oral absorption; 1000 mg orally twice a day for 5 days. It has a more convenient dosage schedule than acyclovir and is approved for adolescents.
- **F. Famciclovir (Famvir)** has a more convenient dosage schedule than acyclovir and is approved for adolescents. Dosage for first episodes of genital HSV infection is 250 mg q8h for 5 days, and for recurrent episodes it is 125 mg twice a day for 5 days.
- **G.** Sexually active individuals known to have genital HSV infection should be advised to use latex condoms even during asymptomatic periods.

References, see page 182.

Urticaria, Angioedema and Anaphylaxis

Urticaria, angioedema, and anaphylaxis are manifestations of the immediate hypersensitivity reaction. Immediate hypersensitivity is an antibody mediated reaction that occurs within minutes to hours of exposure to a particular antigen by an immune individual. Twenty percent of the population will have one of these manifestations, especially urticaria, at some time during life.

- **I. Pathophysiology**
    - **A. Urticaria** (or hives) is an intensely itchy rash that consists of raised, irregularly shaped wheals. The wheals have a blanched center, surrounded by a red flare. Urticaria is caused by histamine release caused by an immunologic reaction between antigens and IgE antibodies. Antigens, chemicals and physical agents (detergents or ultraviolet light) can cause urticaria.
    - **B. Angioedema** is an area of circumscribed swelling of any part of the body. It may be caused by the same mechanisms that cause hives except that the immunologic events occur deeper in the cutis or in the submucosal tissue of the respiratory or gastrointestinal tract.
    - **C. Anaphylaxis** is the acute reaction that occurs when an antigen is introduced systemically into an individual who has preexisting IgE antibodies.
        1. The patient has difficulty breathing from constriction of the major airways and shock due to hypotension caused by histamine release.
        2. Anaphylactoid reactions are not immunologically mediated. Mannitol, radiocontrast material, and drugs (opiates, vancomycin) may degranulate mast cells and cause a reaction that resembles anaphylaxis.

II. Anaphylaxis

A. Causes of anaphylaxis include penicillins, insect venoms, airborne allergens, foods (peanuts, eggs, milk, seafoods, and food dyes and flavors), antitoxins to tetanus, and products of animal origin.

B. Symptoms of anaphylaxis include pruritus, injection of the mucous membranes, bronchospasm, and hypotension.

C. Prevention of anaphylaxis. Anaphylaxis is best prevented by avoidance of the cause. However, anaphylaxis frequently is unanticipated. Individuals with a history of anaphylaxis should be provided with injectable epinephrine. Short-term desensitization may be needed in a patient requiring antibiotic treatment.

D. Treatment of acute anaphylaxis

1. Epinephrine in a 1:1000 dilution (1.0 mg/mL) should be injected at 10-20 min intervals at 0.01 mL/kg SQ per dose, with a maximum dose of 0.3 mL per dose SQ.
2. Oxygen should be administered (100%, 4-6 L/min) and the airway should be secured.
3. Albuterol, 0.1-0.2 mL/kg in a 5 mg/mL solution, should be given via nebulizer every 4-6 hours.
4. Administration of diphenhydramine or chlorpheniramine and corticosteroids should be considered when a complete response to epinephrine does not occur.

III. Urticaria

A. Hives most commonly results from ingestion of foods, food additives, or drugs. These usually cause hive formation for only a few hours to two days. Hives also may be associated with infections caused by parasites or viruses (eg, hepatitis or infectious mononucleosis).

B. Cold urticaria may be induced by exposure to cold, which may result in hypotension after immersion in cold water.

C. Cholinergic urticaria is characterized by the appearance of small punctate wheals, surrounded by a prominent erythematous flare. These small papular urtications are pruritic and appear predominantly on the neck and upper thorax. The lesions often develop after exercise, sweating, exposure to heat, or anxiety. The lesions are caused by stimulation of cholinergic fibers.

D. Solar urticaria may be caused by various wavelengths of light (280-500 nm). It is uncommon, and it is treated with sun screens.

E. Chronic urticaria is caused by ingestion of food substances that contain natural salicylates. Sensitivity to the food additive tartrazine yellow No. 5 frequently is found in patients with salicylate sensitivity.

F. Exercise urticaria is characterized by hives and bronchospasm after exercise.

G. Genetic deficiencies of complement factor H or factor I may cause urticaria. Patients who have these defects frequently develop severe hives, particularly after exposure to cold or hot water or alcohol ingestion.

H. Treatment of urticaria. Urticaria generally is a self-limiting disorder and usually requires only antihistamines. Hydroxyzine 0.5 mg/kg is the most effective treatment. Diphenhydramine 1.25 mg/kg every 6 hrs is also effective.

IV. Angioedema

A. Angioedema is similar to hives, but the reaction occurs deeper in the dermis. It causes diffuse circumscribed swelling. Angioedema is often acquired, or it may be observed in an inherited disease known as hereditary angioneurotic edema (HANE).

B. Hereditary Angioneurotic Edema

1. HANE is characterized by episodes of localized subcutaneous edema of any part of the body.

2. Attacks of severe abdominal cramps and vomiting may be caused by edema of the bowel wall. It may lead to unnecessary surgery if not recognized early. Severe attacks of colic may occur during infancy.

3. Laryngeal edema may sometimes progress to total upper airway obstruction, pulmonary edema, and death. Attacks of palatal and laryngeal edema may follow dental trauma or occur during upper respiratory infections.

4. HANE is inherited as an autosomal dominant disease. It never skips a generation. However, about 10% of cases are caused by new spontaneous mutations, which are passed to offspring.

5. Prophylaxis against attacks of angioedema can be achieved with impeded androgens (ie, androgens that are only minimally virilizing). Stanozolol, at a dose of 2 mg/day; or danazol, 50-300 mg/day, can prevent attacks of angioedema. Other effective maintenance therapies include epsilon amino caproic acid and tranexamic acid. Preparations of C1 inhibitor have been used extensively in Europe.

C. **Acute angioedema** does not generally respond to epinephrine, antihistamines, or steroids. Treatment consists of supportive therapy with IV fluids, analgesics, and airway management. Fresh frozen plasma is generally effective.

References, see page 182.

Infectious Diseases

Fever Without Source in Infants and Young Children

Two-thirds of children visit their physician with an acute febrile illness before the age of three. The most common causes of fever in children are respiratory, urinary tract, gastrointestinal, and central nervous system infections. Bacteremia may occur with any of these infections. Fever without a source that is related to a viral illness is often difficult to differentiate from occult bacteremia.

I. **Clinical evaluation of the febrile child.** The child's health status, course of the current illness, birth and past medical history, and immunization should be evaluated. Infants at risk for serious bacterial infection include those with chronic illness, previous hospitalizations, prematurity, newborn complications, or previous antimicrobial therapy.

II. **Physical examination**
   A. Assessment of cardiopulmonary status includes a determination of vital signs. Children who are toxic require immediate cardiovascular stabilization, a complete sepsis evaluation, and empiric antimicrobial therapy.
   B. Fever is defined as a rectal temperature of at least 38.0°C (100.4°F). Axillary and tympanic measurements are unreliable. Over bundling of small infants can cause temperature elevations. When this is suspected, the temperature should be rechecked with the child unbundled for 15 minutes.
   C. If no focal bacterial infection (eg, skin, soft tissue infection, otitis media) is apparent, the child is at low risk for serious bacterial infection.
   D. **Toxicity** is characterized by signs of sepsis (lethargy, poor perfusion, marked hypoventilation or hyperventilation, or cyanosis). The quality of cry, reaction to parents, color, state of hydration, response to social overtures, affect, respiratory status and effort, and peripheral perfusion should be assessed.
   E. Neonates with acute bacterial meningitis often lack meningismus. Meningitis in neonates may manifest as temperature instability (hyperthermia or hypothermia), poor feeding, listlessness, lethargy, irritability, vomiting, or respiratory distress. A bulging fontanelle may be seen in one-third of cases. The most common CNS signs in the newborn are lethargy and irritability.
   F. In older infants and children, initial symptoms of bacterial meningitis consist of fever, signs of increased intracranial pressure, and cerebral cortical dysfunction. Fever in children who have bacterial meningitis usually is greater than 38.3°C. Increased intracranial pressure may manifest as vomiting and lethargy.
   G. Older children and adolescents frequently present with headache, fever, altered sensorium, and meningismus. Kernig's or Brudzinski's signs may be absent in up to 50% of adolescents and adults with meningitis.

Clinical and Laboratory Findings in Toxic and Non-toxic Infants and Children

Febrile Infants at Low Risk	Toxic Infant or Child
History No previous hospitalizations or chronic illness Term delivery without complications No previous antibiotic therapy **Physical Examination** Nontoxic clinical appearance No focal bacterial infection (except otitis media) Activity, hydration and perfusion normal **Social Situation** Parents/caregiver mature and reliable Thermometer and telephone at child's home **Laboratory Criteria** White blood cell count of 5,000-15,000/mm³ Band cell count <1,500/mm³ Normal urinalysis (<5 white blood cells/high-power field) When diarrhea is present, less than 5 white blood cells/high-power field in stool	Slow, irregular or decreasing respiratory rate Head bobbing Stridor Paradoxic or abdominal breathing Chest retractions Central cyanosis Altered level of consciousness Fever with petechiae Tachypnea Grunting Prolonged expiration Nasal flaring Poor muscle tone Poor or delayed capillary refill Tachycardia

Normal Pediatric Vital Signs

Age	Respiratory Rate (breaths per minute)	Heart Rate (beats per minute)	Systolic Blood Pressure	Diastolic Blood pressure
Newborn	40-60	90-170	50-92	25-45
One month	30-50	110-180	60-104	20-60
Six months	25-35	110-180	65-125	53-66
One year	20-30	80-160	70-118	53-66
Two years	20-30	80-130	70-117	53-66
Three years	20-30	80-120	70-117	53-66

III. Laboratory studies
   A. Reassuring laboratory screening values include a white blood cell count of 5,000 to 15,000/mm³ (5.0 to 15.0 x 10/L), an absolute band cell count of <1,500/mm³, and fewer than 5 white blood cells per high-power field in stool specimens in infants with diarrhea.
   B. **Gram-stained smear of urine sediment** is a sensitive screening test; a urine

culture should be obtained to confirm urinary tract infection.

C. **Blood cultures** are valuable in confirming bacteremia.

D. **Lumbar puncture** is mandatory when the diagnosis of meningitis is suspected in a febrile child because it is the only test that can exclude this diagnosis.

IV. **Management of fever without source**

A. **Toxic-appearing infants and children**

1. All toxic-appearing febrile infants and children less than 36 months of age should be hospitalized for evaluation and treatment of meningitis or possible sepsis.

2. Occult bacteremia can lead to osteomyelitis, septic arthritis, meningitis, urinary tract infection, pneumonia, enteritis, and meningitis.

B. **Febrile infants less than 28 days of age**

1. Fever in infants less than 28 days of age always mandates a sepsis evaluation and hospitalization for parenteral antibiotic therapy until culture results are known.

2. Laboratory evaluation includes an examination of cerebrospinal fluid for cells, glucose, protein and culture; a urinalysis and urine culture; and a blood culture.

C. **Febrile infants 28 to 90 days of age**

1. Infants who do not meet low-risk criteria should be hospitalized for a sepsis evaluation and empiric antimicrobial therapy until culture results are known.

2. Febrile infants less than three months of age who meet low-risk criteria, can be observed after a urine culture has been obtained.

3. Empiric parenteral antimicrobial therapy may be used in the outpatient management of low-risk infants. Ceftriaxone (Rocephin), a third-generation parenteral cephalosporin with a half-life of 5-6 hours, is often used; 50 mg/kg once daily.

4. Children who have met low-risk criteria with reliable parents can be treated as outpatients if close follow-up within 18-24 hours can be ensured. Caregivers are instructed to check the child every 4 hours for activity, rectal temperature, and skin color.

D. **Febrile children 3 months to 36 months of age**

1. Occult bacteremia in febrile children 3 to 36 months of age without a source of infection has an incidence of 3-11%, with a mean probability of 4.3% in children with a temperature of at least 39.0°C (102.2°F). The risk of bacteremia correlates with the height of the fever.

2. Nontoxic-appearing children with a fever of less than 39.0°C (102.2°F), who have been previously healthy, may be managed expectantly if there is no apparent focus of infection. Acetaminophen, 15 mg/kg/dose q4h, is given for fever, and the child is reevaluated if the fever persists for more than 48 hours or if the child's clinical condition worsens.

3. Children with a fever greater than 39.0°C (102.2°F) may require a lumbar puncture, white blood cell count, and empiric antimicrobial therapy.

   a. Children with a white blood cell count of 15,000/mm^3 or more require a blood culture and treatment with empiric antimicrobial therapy.

   b. Children with a white blood cell count of less than 15,000/mm^3 and a benign clinical appearance can be managed expectantly with antipyretics and return of the child if fever persists for more than 48 hours or if the child's clinical condition worsens.

References, see page 182.

Bacterial Meningitis

Bacterial meningitis affects 1 in 500 children younger than 2 years. Meningitis most commonly presents with subtle signs and symptoms that may easily be mistaken for a benign childhood illness.

I. **Etiology of Bacterial Meningitis**
   A. **Neonatal Meningitis – 0 to 3 Months of Age**
      1. The most common bacterial agents responsible for CNS infection in infants 0 to 3 months of life (in declining order of frequency) are: group B *Streptococcus* (GBS), *Escherichia coli*, *Listeria*, *Enterococcus*, Gram-negative enteric bacilli other than *E coli*, fungi, and anaerobes.
      2. The preterm infant is considered an immunocompromised host; thus, all agents should be considered, including bacteria, viruses, *Mycoplasma*, *Ureaplasma*, and fungi, as potential causes of CNS infection in this group.

Common Etiologic Agents of Meningitis by Age Group				
Organism	**0-3 Months**	**3-36 Months**	**3-21 Years**	**Immunoco mpromised**
Group B Streptococcus	X			
Escherichia coli	X			
Listeria monocytogenes	X			
Streptococcus pneumoniae		X	X	X
Neisseria meningitidis		X	X	X
Fungus				X
Cryptococcus				X
Tuberculosis		X		
Virus	X	X	X	X

Note: Haemophilus influenzae no longer is a common pathogen in countries where the conjugate vaccines are used routinely.

   B. **Infancy – 3 Months to 3 Years**. Since the advent and increased use of the *Haemophilus* conjugate vaccines, the principal causes of bacterial meningitis in this age group are *N meningitidis* and *S pneumoniae*.
   C. **Childhood – 3 to 21 Years**. The most common bacterial agents for meningitis in this age group are *N meningitidis* and *S pneumoniae*. Viral meningitis, principally caused by the enteroviruses, arboviruses, and herpesviruses, account for most of the CNS disease in this age group.

II. **Clinical evaluation**
   A. **Signs and symptoms** of meningitis include fever, headache, neck pain or

stiffness, nausea, vomiting, photophobia, and irritability. Young infants may exhibit only signs of irritability, somnolence, and low-grade fever. Meningitis always must be considered in any young infant whose temperature is greater than 38.2°C (100.7°F) and who has no obvious site of infection.

B. **Physical findings** include lethargy, somnolence, stiff neck, rash, petechia, purpura, and hemodynamic instability.

C. **Lumbar puncture** remains the most important early diagnostic test. Rapid antigen testing of the CSF and urine are specific but not sensitive indicators of disease; with the exception of *Haemophilus* meningitis, it rarely provides helpful information in guiding initial therapy.

D. **Gram stain** of a CSF smear is very helpful. CSF protein levels greater than 100 to 120 mg/dL are suggestive of bacterial meningitis.

E. **Culture** remains the standard for diagnosis of meningitis. Blood culture, Gram stain of a CSF smear, CSF culture, urinalysis, and urine culture should be performed routinely in all children who are suspected of having meningitis.

Cerebrospinal Fluid Findings in Normal and Infected Hosts					
Disorder	**Color**	**WBC Count (/mm³)**	**Glucose (mg/dL)**	**Protein (mg/dL)**	**Gram's Stain and culture**
Normal infant	clear	<10	>40	90	negative
Normal child or adult	clear	0	>40	<40	negative
Bacterial meningitis	cloudy	200-10000	<40	100-500	usually positive
Viral meningitis	clear	25-1000 (<50% PMN)	>40	50-100	negative

F. **CSF analysis** must include cell count, differential, and protein and glucose concentrations. If the CSF indices suggest viral, fungal, or tuberculous disease, specific stains and cultures should be requested. When viral meningitis is suspected, rectal swabs, CSF and peripheral buffy coat viral cultures, and PCR should be considered. For the immunocompromised patient, cryptococcal antigen or an India ink-stained smear of CSF provides quick identification.

G. Complete blood count, platelet count, and serum electrolyte concentrations are helpful as baseline studies. The syndrome of inappropriate antidiuretic hormone (SIADH) occurs in 30-60% of children who have bacterial meningitis. Seizures occur in 20% to 30% of patients before or during the first 3 days after diagnosis of meningitis.

III. Management of bacterial meningitis

A. Term infants in the first month of life are treated with a combination of ampicillin with either gentamicin or cefotaxime. For low-birthweight preterm infants in the nursery who present with late-onset meningitis, an antistaphylococcal agent such as methicillin or vancomycin and an aminoglycoside are used until culture results are available.

B. Infants 1 to 2 months of age are treated with ampicillin and cefotaxime or ampicillin and ceftriaxone, which provide coverage against enterococci and *Listeria* as well as the normal pathogens beyond the newborn period.

C. Infants and children older than 2 months of age. Resistant strains of *S pneumoniae* have become a major problem among. Initial meningitis therapy must include vancomycin in dosages of 60 mg/kg per day in four divided doses in addition to either cefotaxime or ceftriaxone. This dosage of vancomycin should be adjusted to maintain peak serum concentrations of 30 to 40 mcg/mL and trough values of 5 to 10 mcg/mL. The initial dosage of cefotaxime is 75 mg/kg per dose every 6 hours. Ceftriaxone dosage is 80 to 100 mg/kg daily in one dose; an extra dose is given on the first day at 12 hours.

Dosages of Antibiotics Administered Intravenously to Newborn Infants and Children

Antibiotic	Age (Days)	Dosage	Desired Serum Concentrations (Mcg/ml)
Ampicillin	0-7 7-30 >30	50 mg/kg/dose q8h 50-75 mg/kg/dose q6h 50-75 q6h	Not critical to measure
Cefotaxime (Claforan)	0-7 7-30 >30	50 mg/kg/dose q8h 50-75 mg/kg/dose q6h 75 q6h	Not critical to measure
Ceftriaxone (Rocephin)	All	80-100 mg/kg/dose. At diagnosis, 12 h, 24 h, and every 24 h thereafter	Not critical to measure
Gentamicin	0-7 7-30 >30	2.5 mg/kg/dose q12h 2.5 mg/kg/dose q8h 2.5 mg/kg/dose q8h	Peak, 6-10 Trough,<2
Vancomycin	0-7 7-30 >30	15 mg/kg/dose q12h 15 mg/kg/dose q8h 15 mg/kg/dose q6h	Peak, 30-40 Trough, 5-10

D. Dexamethasone. If CSF indices suggest bacterial meningitis or if organisms are seen on Gram stain of a CSF smear, dexamethasone is recommended in a dosage of 0.6 mg/kg per day in two to four divided doses for 2 to 4 days. The initial dose of steroid should be infused before the initial dose of parenteral antibiotics.

References, see page 182.

Otitis Media

Otitis media is the most commonly diagnosed illness in childhood. This infection occurs in half of all infants before their first birthday and in 80% by their third birthday. Half of all infected children will have 3 or more episodes in their first 3 years of life.

I. **Pathophysiology**
   A. Otitis media is classified as either acute otitis media or otitis media with effusion.
   B. **Acute otitis media** consists of inflammation of the middle ear, presenting with a rapid onset of symptoms and clinical signs of ear pathology. Fever and ear pain are the most common acute symptoms. Irritability, anorexia, vomiting, and diarrhea may also be present. Acute otitis media is most common in children 6 months to 3 years. The majority of children have had at least one episode of acute otitis by age 3. It is uncommon after age 8. The incidence rises during winter and declines during summer.
   C. **Otitis media with effusion** consists of a chronic bacterial infection persisting more than 2 weeks, manifesting as an asymptomatic middle-ear effusion. The syndrome usually develops after an acute otitis media.

II. **Microbiology**
   A. **Common pathogens.** The most common bacterial pathogen in all age groups is Streptococcus pneumoniae, causing 40% of effusions. The next most common is non-typable Haemophilus influenzae, causing 20% of effusions. Anaerobic bacteria, Chlamydia or Mycoplasma cause less than 2-5%.
   B. **Ampicillin resistence** caused by beta-lactamase occurs in 30-50% of H influenzae and up to 80% of M. catarrhalis.
   C. **Penicillin-resistant S. pneumoniae** results from bacterial alterations in penicillin-binding proteins, rather than beta-lactamase. Highly resistant strains are resistant to penicillin, trimethoprim/sulfamethoxazole (TMP/SMX), and third-generation cephalosporins. The prevalence of multiple-drug resistant S. pneumoniae is 20-35%.

III. **Diagnosis**
   A. **Acute otitis media**
      1. The position, color, translucency and mobility of the tympanic membrane should be assessed. The normal eardrum is translucent, and landmarks should be visible through the eardrum. A cloudy opacified tympanic membrane in children is often associated with a middle ear effusion. Erythema of the eardrum alone is often the result of a viral infection or crying.
      2. Reduced or absent mobility of the tympanic membrane with air insufflation is the most specific sign of acute otitis media.
      3. In otitis media, the tympanic membrane is dull and bulges externally, losing its concave contour and light reflex. An air-fluid level or air bubbles may sometimes be visualized behind the tympanic membrane.
   B. **Otitis media with effusion**
      1. In the absence of symptoms or signs of acute illness, evidence of middle

ear inflammation indicates that an otitis media with effusion is present. Typical findings include diminished tympanic membrane mobility and visualization of air-fluid levels.

2. The sensation of fullness in the ear or obvious hearing loss may be present.

IV. Treatment of acute otitis media

A. First-line antibiotics

1. Oral antibiotics should be prescribed for 10-14 days.

2. **Amoxicillin** is the first-line antimicrobial agent for treating AOM, at doses of 80-90 mg/kg/d. For patients with treatment failure after three days of therapy, alternative agents include oral amoxicillin-clavulanate, cefuroxime axetil, and intramuscular ceftriaxone.

3. **Streptococcus pneumoniae** causes 40-50% of all cases of AOM. This agent has reduced susceptibility to penicillin in 8-35% (2-4% highly resistant) of isolates and reduced susceptibility to third-generation cephalosporins in 10% of isolates (about 4% highly resistant).

4. **Cefuroxime axetil (Ceftin) and amoxicillin-clavulanate (Augmentin) orally, and ceftriaxone (Rocephin)** intramuscularly, are useful as second-line drugs for treatment failure, which is defined as ear pain, fever, or bulging tympanic membrane or otorrhea after three days of therapy.

5. Trimethoprim-sulfamethoxazole, erythromycin-sulfisoxazole, clarithromycin and azithromycin are ineffective for AOM.

Second-Line Antibiotic Therapy for Acute Otitis Media		
Drug	Dosage	Comments
Amoxicillin-clavulanic acid (Augmentin)	40 mg/kg of amoxicillin component in 3 divided doses	Diarrhea common
Cefuroxime axetil (Ceftin)	500 mg in 2 divided doses	
Ceftriaxone (Rocephin)	50 mg/kg	

References, see page 182.

Pneumonia

A lower respiratory tract infection (LRI) develops in one in three children in the first year of life. Twenty-nine percent of these children develop pneumonia, 15% develop croup, 34% tracheobronchitis, and 29% bronchiolitis.

I. Clinical evaluation of pneumonia

A. Cough. Pneumonia usually causes cough that persists day and night. Patients who cough spontaneously throughout the office visit are likely to have lower respiratory tract disease.

B. Grunting occurs in 20% of infants who have bronchiolitis or pneumonia. Grunting prevents collapse of narrowed airways and improves oxygenation.

C. Chest pain. Pneumonia causes chest pain when the infection develops near the pleura. Pneumonia that involves the diaphragmatic pleura may present as abdominal pain. Older children may complain of diffuse chest or abdominal pain, which is caused by persistent cough and repeated muscle contraction.

D. **Tachypnea**. Increased respiratory rate is one of the earliest and most consistent signs of lower respiratory tract disease.

Abnormal Respiratory Rates by Age	
Age	Abnormal
<2 months	>60 bpm
2-12 months old	>50 bpm
>1 year old	>40 bpm

E. **Retractions.** Retractions of the intercostal spaces may occur with pneumonia because of decreased compliance or increased airway resistance.

F. **Auscultation**
   1. **Signs of consolidation** include dullness to percussion and increased transmission of the voice on auscultation.
   2. **Crackles** are the fine popping sounds that occur when previously closed airways open suddenly. They indicate pulmonary parenchymal disease.
   3. **Wheezing** is generated by narrowed airways. It can be caused by bronchiolitis, asthma, early pulmonary edema, subglottic stenosis, or tracheal compression.

G. **Cyanosis** occurs at an oxygen saturation of 67%; however, cyanosis will not manifest in the presence of anemia. It is not a sensitive predictor of pneumonia because significantly hypoxemia may be present before cyanosis is visible.

II. **Diagnostic evaluation of lower respiratory infections**
   A. **Chest radiograph.** A chest radiograph should be obtained when pneumonia fails to improve on antibiotics, or when the child appears acutely ill.
   B. **Laboratory tests**
      1. **WBC count** should be obtained for children who have significant fever (>38°C in infants, >39°C in children), who appear ill, or who are hospitalized.
      2. **Blood cultures** are rarely positive in children with pneumonia. They should be obtained in infants and children with high fever, ill appearance, or upon hospitalization.
      3. **Bacterial antigen assays** of urine by latex agglutination, or antibody tests of blood influence therapy only rarely with unusual infections or when pneumonia is unresponsive to therapy.
      4. **Nasopharyngeal cultures for viruses** and immunofluorescence studies for viral antigens are obtained when therapy with antiviral agents is being considered.

III. **Pneumonia in newborns**
   A. Group B streptococcal disease is the most common cause of pneumonia in the newborn. The infection usually is acquired in utero. Prenatal screening of expectant mothers and intrapartum prophylaxis of colonized mothers with IV ampicillin decreases the incidence.
   B. Initial therapy of pneumonia in newborns consists of ampicillin (100 mg/kg IV initial dose, followed by 200 mg/kg/day divided QID) and gentamicin (2.5 mg/kg

IV initial dose, followed by 7.5 mg/kg/day divided q8h).

Management of Pneumonia in Children					
Patient	Chest Radiograph	Blood Count	Blood Gas	Blood Culture	Antibiotics
Newborn	+	+	+	+	Ampicillin and gentamicin
Infant Febrile/Ill-appearing	+	+	+	+	Nafcillin and cefotaxime
Afebrile/Well-appearing	+	+	±	-	Erythromycin or clarithromycin PO
Toddler Febrile/ill-appearing	+	+	+	+	Amoxicillin or cefuroxime
Afebrile/Well-appearing	+	±	+	+	None (close follow-up)
Child Febrile/ill-appearing	+	+	±	±	Cefuroxime
Afebrile/Well-appearing	+				Erythromycin or clarithromycin PO

IV. **Pneumonia in infants (2 weeks to 6 months)**
   A. **Febrile/ill-appearing infants**
      1. Pathogens in this age group include Streptococcus pneumoniae and Haemophilus influenzae serotype B (HIB). HIB has all but disappeared because of vaccination. Staphylococcus aureus is also a potential pathogen, which frequently causes pleural effusion (55%) or pneumothorax (21%).
      2. Evaluation of the ill-appearing, febrile infant for sepsis includes blood cultures, urine culture, chest radiograph, complete blood count, and a lumbar puncture.
      3. Initial parenteral antibiotic therapy consists of nafcillin (100-150 mg/kg/day divided QID) to cover staphylococci, and cefotaxime (100-150 mg/kg/day divided TID) for Gram-negative pathogens. Alternative therapy is cefuroxime (100-150 mg/kg/day divided TID).
   B. **Afebrile/well-appearing infants**
      1. In infants with afebrile pneumonia, the pathogens most commonly are Chlamydia trachomatis (25%), Ureaplasma urealyticum (21%), cytomegalovirus (20%), and Pneumocystis carinii (18%).
      2. Chlamydia antigens can be detected by direct flourescent antibody and enzyme-linked immunoassay techniques.
      3. RSV, adenovirus, and the parainfluenza viruses also can cause pneu-

monia in otherwise well infants. Viral antigen detection kits are available for these common viral pathogens.

4. Bordetella pertussis infection may cause paroxysms of cough in an otherwise well-appearing infant. The characteristic "whoop" cough is not always present.

5. Infants with afebrile pneumonia are treated as outpatients. Hospitalization is required for infants with inability to eat, respiratory distress, or hypoxemia. Erythromycin (50 mg/kg/day divided QID) or clarithromycin [(Biaxin) 15 mg/kg/day PO bid] are drugs of choice.

V. Pneumonia in toddlers and preschoolers

A. Afebrile/well-appearing toddlers and preschoolers

1. The majority of pneumonia among in this age group is caused by viral infection with RSV, parainfluenza, adenovirus, or influenza, or by other viruses (enterovirus, rhinovirus), or Mycoplasma pneumoniae.

2. A chest radiograph is usually not necessary. This pneumonia can usually be treated symptomatically, without antibiotic therapy.

B. Febrile/ill-appearing Toddlers and Preschoolers

1. Pneumococcus is the most common bacterial pathogen causing febrile pneumonia in children and adults. The syndrome is characterized by acute onset of high, spiking fever, with chills, cough and sputum production. Crackles may be heard on auscultation, leukocytosis is frequent, and the chest radiograph will demonstrate lobar pneumonia.

2. Neisseria meningitidis infection also may present with febrile pneumonia; however, signs of meningococcemia, such as petechiae and sepsis syndrome, are usually present.

3. Outpatient therapy is appropriate for otherwise healthy, alert, cooperative children. Pneumococcus usually is sensitive to amoxicillin (40 mg/kg/day divided TID).

4. If the patient does not tolerate oral medication, intramuscular ceftriaxone (50 mg/kg with lidocaine) may be given initially.

5. Severely ill patients (ie, hypoxemia, respiratory insufficiency) require parenteral therapy. Intravenous ampicillin (100 mg/kg/day divided QID) is initiated. Cefuroxime (150 mg/kg/day divided TID) is an acceptable alternative. If hypoxemia is present, oxygen is given by nasal cannula.

VI. Pneumonia in children and adolescents

A. Atypical bacteria, Mycoplasma pneumoniae and C pneumoniae, are responsible for a significant proportion of afebrile lower respiratory tract disease in adolescents and school-age children.

B. Atypical pneumonia may be associated with a prodrome of headache and abdominal symptoms. Onset usually is insidious with low-grade fever.

C. These bacteria are susceptible to erythromycin. The recommended dose of the estolate form (Ilosone) is 30-40 mg/kg/day divided q8-12 hours. If GI upset occurs, a lower dose can be used or the drug can be administered after clear liquids or crackers.

D. Clarithromycin (Biaxin), 15 mg/kg/day PO bid, is also effective against these pathogens. Tetracycline (25-50 mg/kg/day divided QID) and doxycycline (2-4 mg/kg/day divided BID) also are effective against Mycoplasma and Chlamydia and can be used in children older than 8 years.

References, see page 182.

Bronchiolitis

Bronchiolitis is an acute wheezing-associated illness which occurs in early life, preceded by signs and symptoms of an upper respiratory infection. Infants may have a single episode of bronchiolitis or may have multiple occurrences in the first year of life.

I. **Epidemiology**
   A. Bronchiolitis occurs most frequently from early November and continues through April.
   B. Bronchiolitis is most serious in infants who are less than one year old, especially those 1-3 months old. Infants at risk include those who are raised in crowded living conditions, who are passively exposed to tobacco smoke, and who are not breast-fed.

II. **Pathophysiology**
   A. Respiratory syncytial virus (RSV) is the leading cause of bronchiolitis in infants and young children, accounting for 50% of cases of bronchiolitis requiring hospitalization.
   B. Infants born prematurely, or with bronchopulmonary dysplasia (BPD), immunodeficiency or congenital heart disease are at especially high risk for severe RSV illness.
   C. RSV is transmitted by contact with nasal secretions. Shedding of virus occurs 1 to 2 days before symptoms occur, and for 1 to 2 weeks afterwards. Symptoms usually last an average of 5 days.
   D. Parainfluenza viruses are the second most frequent cause of bronchiolitis. They cause illness during autumn and spring, before and after outbreaks of RSV. Influenza A virus, adenovirus, rhinovirus and Mycoplasma pneumonia can all cause bronchiolitis. Rhinovirus and mycoplasma pneumonia cause wheezing-associated respiratory illness in older children, while parainfluenza virus and RSV can cause wheezing at any age.
   E. Bacterial agents almost never cause bronchiolitis. Superinfection with bacteria is rare in cases of RSV bronchiolitis.

III. **Clinical evaluation of bronchiolitis**
   A. Symptoms of RSV may range from those of a mild cold to severe bronchiolitis or pneumonia. RSV infection frequently begins with nasal discharge, pharyngitis, and cough. Hoarseness or laryngitis is not common. Fever occurs in most young children, with temperatures ranging from 38°°C to 40°°C (100.4°°F to 104°°F). The respiratory rate may be remarkably elevated, often reaching 80 breaths/min.
   B. **Hyperresonance of the chest wall** may be present, and wheezing can be heard in most infants without auscultation. The wheezing sound is harsh and low in pitch, although severely affected infants may not have detectable wheezing at the time of the examination. Fine "crackles" are usually heard on inspiration. Substernal and intercostal retractions are often noted.
   C. **Cyanosis** of the oral mucosa and nail beds may occur in severely ill infants. Restlessness and hyperinflation of the chest wall are signs of impending respiratory failure.

IV. **Diagnosis**
   A. Infants with bronchiolitis present symptoms of an upper respiratory illness for several days and wheezing during the peak RSV season.
   B. **Chest radiography** typically shows hyperexpansion and diffuse interstitial pneumonitis. Consolidation is noted in about 25% of children, most commonly

in the right upper or middle lobe.

C. **Oxygen saturation** values of <95% suggest the need for hospitalization.

D. **Arterial blood gases** should be obtained to assess the severity of respiratory compromise. Carbon dioxide levels are commonly in the 30-35 mm Hg range. Respiratory failure is suggested by CO_2 values of 45-55 mm Hg. Arterial O_2 indicates severe disease, especially when the O_2 tension drops below 66 mm Hg.

E. **White blood cell count** may be normal or elevated slightly, and the differential count may show neutrophilia.

F. **Enzyme-linked immunosorbent assays** (ELISA) of nasal washings for RSV are highly sensitive and specific.

V. **Management**

A. Outpatient management of bronchiolitis is appropriate for infants with mild disease.

B. **Criteria for hospitalization**
1. History of prematurity (especially less than 34 weeks)
2. Congenital heart disease
3. Other underlying lung disease
4. Low initial oxygen saturation suggestive of respiratory failure (O_2 saturation <95%, with a toxic, distressed appearance)
5. Age ≤3 months
6. Dehydrated infant who is not feeding well
7. Unreliable parents

C. Before hospitalization, infants should receive an aerosolized beta-adrenergic agent. A few infants will respond to this therapy and avoid hospitalization. If the response is good, the infant can be sent home, and an oral albuterol continued.

D. Hospitalized infants should receive hydration and ambient oxygen to maintain an oxygen saturation ≥92-93% by pulse oximetry.

E. **Treatment of bronchiolitis in the hospital**
1. **Racemic epinephrine by inhalation** may be administered as a therapeutic trial. It should be continued if an improvement in the respiratory status is noted.
2. **Ribavirin**
a. Ribavirin, an antiviral agent, produces modest improvement in clinical illness and oxygenation. Ribavirin is helpful in severely ill or high-risk patients.

Indications for Ribavirin Use in Bronchiolitis	
Congenital heart disease, especially cyanotic	Immunodeficiency due to chemotherapy
Bronchopulmonary dysplasia	Cystic fibrosis
Renal transplantation, recent	Severe combined immunodeficiency
Age <6 weeks	Multiple congenital anomalies
Neurologic diseases	Certain premature infants
Heart failure of any cause	Metabolic diseases
RSV bronchiolitis and arterial O_2 <65 mmHg	RSV bronchiolitis and a rising PCO_2

b. High-dose ribavirin is given for 2 hours, three times a day using an oxygen hood.

c. Treatment with ribavirin combined with RSV immune globulin administered either parenterally or by aerosol is more effective than therapy with either agent alone. Corticosteroid use in the treatment of bronchiolitis is not recommended.

F. Prevention of RSV bronchiolitis with immunoglobulin prophylaxis
1. **Prophylactically administered immunoglobulin with antibody to RSV (RespiGam)** has been shown to reduce the incidence of severe disease and hospitalization in high-risk children. The decision to use RSV-IGIV should be individualized based on risk.

Recommendations for RSV-IGIV Prophylaxis

- ≤2 years old, bronchopulmonary dysplasia, oxygen therapy within 6 months of RSV season.
- ≤28 weeks gestation: up to 12 months of age.
- 29-32 wks gestation: up to 6 months of age.
- Administered monthly during RSV season, usually November to April
- Dose: 750 mg/kg IV
- Immunization with MMR should be varicella deferred for 9 mos.

---

2. Children with cyanotic congenital heart disease are also at significant risk for severe RSV illness and associated mortality.
3. RSV-IGIV, 750 mg/kg, is effective in reducing the severity of RSV infection and the need for and duration of hospitalization of infants at high risk for severe RSV illness.

References, see page 182.

Tonsillopharyngitis

Among uncomplicated cases of upper respiratory tract infections, it is usually important only to identify those children who have a group A streptococcal infection.

I. Classification of acute upper respiratory infections
  A. Among patients who have an uncomplicated acute URI, the most important step is to identify those who do not need an antibiotic from those who have a streptococcal infection and require specific treatment.
  B. Some patients who do not require an antibiotic can be recognized clinically. Such symptoms as rhinitis, conjunctivitis, and cough or the finding of an enanthem or exanthem indicative of an enteroviral infection are indications of respiratory virus infection.
II. Etiology of tonsillopharyngitis
  A. Viruses
    1. The adenoviruses are the most common cause of tonsillopharyngitis, especially types 1, 2, 3, and 5, which are the types that infect small children most frequently. Other respiratory viruses are less common causes of tonsillitis; the parainfluenza viruses probably are the most frequently isolated in this group.
    2. The most frequent causes of the common cold, the rhinoviruses and coronaviruses, involve the tonsils and pharynx less commonly.
  B. Bacteria. Group A Streptococcus is the most important and frequent cause of

tonsillopharyngitis. It is frequently associated with acute rheumatic fever and acute glomerulonephritis. Appropriate treatment of streptococcal pharyngotonsillitis prevents the occurrence of rheumatic fever.

Bacterial Causes of Tonsillopharyngitis in Children

Common
Group A *Streptococcus*

Less Common
Arcanobacterium hemolyticum
Chlamydia pneumoniae
Groups C & G streptococci
Mycoplasma pneumoniae

Unusual
Neisseria gonorrhoeae
N meningitidis

Not causative
C trachomatous
Haemophilus influenzae
Moraxella catarrhalis
Staphylococcus aureus
Streptococcus pneumoniae

III. **Epidemiology**
   A. **Prevalence.** The average incidence of all acute URIs is five to seven per child per year. Group A streptococci is isolated in 30-36.8% of children with pharyngitis.
   B. **Age occurrence.** Pharyngitis is infrequent in the first 2 years of life. Most cases of pharyngitis occur in school-age children, when the incidence of all infections is still high but less than in the first 2 years.
   C. **Etiology**
      1. Viruses are isolated in about 50% of children less than 2 years old but infrequently thereafter.
      2. Group A streptococcus is isolated most frequently in school-age children, while M pneumoniae is found most often in teenagers.
   D. **Season.** Group A Streptococcus causes infections most frequently in late winter and early spring, and it is rare in late spring and summer, although it causes some infections throughout the year.
IV. **Clinical features**
   A. **Bacterial infections**. Only one-third to one-half of patients infected with group A streptococci have classic findings of streptococcal tonsillopharyngitis; the remainder have mild, atypical, or asymptomatic disease.

Features of Streptococcal Tonsillopharyngitis

Sudden onset
Sore throat (pain on swallowing)
Fever
Headache
Nausea, vomiting, abdominal pain (especially in children)
Marked inflammation of throat and tonsils
Patchy discrete exudate
Tender, enlarged anterior cervical nodes
Scarlet fever

Features rarely associated with streptococcal tonsillopharyngitis--suggestive of other etiologies

    Conjunctivitis
    Cough
    Laryngitis (stridor, croup)
    Diarrhea
    Nasal discharge (except in young children)
    Muscle aches/malaise

  B. Viral infections
     1. The adenoviruses are the cause of pharyngoconjunctival fever. Hand, foot, and mouth disease and lymphonodular pharyngitis are caused by the enteroviruses.
     2. The classic feature of herpes simplex infections in young children is gingivostomatitis, but in older children this agent causes tonsillopharyngitis, which is indistinguishable from streptococcal pharyngitis.

V. Laboratory diagnosis
  A. Streptococcal infections
     1. Rapid identification of streptococcal antigens (the rapid strep test) identifies group A streptococcus. When compared with the "gold standard" for the diagnosis of streptococcal pharyngitis--a throat culture--rapid strep tests is specific but not as sensitive.
     2. If a patient has a URI suggestive of streptococcal pharyngitis, a rapid strep test is recommended. If it is positive, one can be certain that there are group A streptococci present in the pharynx. If it is negative, however, a throat culture should be obtained and antibiotics should be initiated while throat culture results are pending. The throat swab should not be placed in a liquid carrier medium after the culture is taken, nor should it be placed in the refrigerator.

VI. Treatment of tonsillopharyngitis
  A. Group A streptococcal infections
     1. Treatment of streptococcal tonsillopharyngitis hastens clinical recovery, makes the patient noninfectious, and prevents suppurative complications and rheumatic fever.
     2. Penicillin is the drug of choice for streptococcal pharyngitis because it has been shown to be effective in preventing rheumatic fever, penicillin-resistant streptococci have not been described, it is inexpensive, and it is relatively nontoxic and safe.
     3. Patients should be treated by one of the following regimens:
       a. Oral penicillin (40 mg/kg/d qid) for 10 days is the drug of choice; erythromycin may be used for patients who have penicillin allergies; other macrolides appear to be effective as well. Other options are

clindamycin or one of the cephalosporins.
- **b.** Intramuscular benzathine penicillin G is used when noncompliance is likely, but is used infrequently in practice because injections are painful.
- **c.** Ineffective antimicrobials include tetracyclines, sulfonamides, and trimethoprim/sulfamethoxazole.
- **B. Follow-up and management of contacts**. Patients become noninfectious rapidly after onset of therapy. They should be sent back to child care, school, or work when they feel well enough.

References, see page 182.

Acute Conjunctivitis

Conjunctivitis is defined as inflammation of the conjunctiva; it is usually caused by infection or allergy. It is often referred to as "pink eye."

- **I. Etiology**
  - **A.** Neonatal conjunctivitis occurs in 1.6-12% of newborns. The most common cause is chemical irritation from antimicrobial prophylaxis against bacterial infection, followed by Chlamydia trachomatis infection. Haemophilus influenzae and Streptococcus pneumoniae may also cause infection in newborns.
  - **B.** Rarely, gram-negative organisms such as Escherichia coli, Klebsiella, or Pseudomonas sp can cause neonatal conjunctivitis. Neisseria gonorrhoeae is an unusual cause of neonatal conjunctivitis because of the use of ocular prophylaxis.
  - **C.** Herpes simplex can cause neonatal keratoconjunctivitis; however, it is almost always associated with infection of the skin and mucous membranes, or with disseminated disease. The presence of vesicles anywhere on the body in association with neonatal conjunctivitis is suggestive of herpes.
  - **D.** In older infants and children, H influenzae is by far the most common identifiable cause of conjunctivitis, causing 40-50% of episodes. S pneumoniae accounts for 10% of cases, and Moraxella catarrhalis is the third most common cause. Chlamydia trachomatis can rarely cause conjunctivitis in sexually active adolescents.
  - **E.** Adenovirus is the most important viral cause of acute conjunctivitis. This organism often causes epidemics of acute conjunctivitis. It causes 20% of childhood conjunctivitis (most occurring in the fall and winter months).
- **II. Clinical presentation**
  - **A. In the first day of life**, conjunctivitis is usually caused by chemical conjunctivitis secondary to ocular prophylaxis.
  - **B. Three to 5 days after birth**, gonococcal conjunctivitis is the most common cause of conjunctivitis.
  - **C. After the first week of life and throughout the first month**, chlamydia is the most frequent cause of conjunctivitis, presenting with hyperemia. Severe cases are associated with a thick mucopurulent discharge and pseudomembrane formation.
  - **D.** Gonococcal conjunctivitis can present as typical bacterial conjunctivitis, or as a hyperacute conjunctivitis with profuse purulent discharge. There often is severe edema of both lids.
  - **E.** In the older infant and child, both viral and bacterial conjunctivitis may present with an acutely inflamed eye. Typically, there is conjunctival erythema, with

occasional lid edema. Exudate often accumulates during the night. Bacterial conjunctivitis tends to be more common in the preschooler and is more likely to be bilateral and associated with an exudate than is viral conjunctivitis.

F. Many patients who have both adenoviral conjunctivitis and pharyngitis also are febrile. The triad of pharyngitis, conjunctivitis, and fever has been termed pharyngoconjunctival fever.

III. Diagnosis

A. Neonates

1. In cases of neonatal conjunctivitis, a Gram stain and culture should be obtained to exclude N gonorrhoeae conjunctivitis.
2. Chlamydia trachomatis antigen detection assays have a sensitivity and specificity of 90% or better.

B. Infants and older children.
Outside the neonatal period, a Gram stain is usually not needed unless the conjunctivitis lasts longer than 7 days. The presence of vesicles or superficial corneal ulcerations suggests herpetic keratoconjunctivitis.

IV. Differential diagnosis of conjunctivitis

A. Systemic diseases.
Most cases of red eye in children are caused by acute conjunctivitis, allergy, or trauma; however, Kawasaki disease, Lyme disease, leptospirosis, juvenile rheumatoid arthritis, and Stevens-Johnson syndrome may cause conjunctivitis. Glaucoma is a significant cause of a red eye in adults; however, it is rare in children.

B. Allergic conjunctivitis

1. Allergic eye disease is characterized by pronounced ocular itching, redness, tearing, and photophobia. This recurrent disease has seasonal exacerbations in the spring, summer, and fall. Children who have allergic conjunctivitis often have other atopic diseases (rhinitis, eczema, asthma) and a positive family history. Allergic conjunctivitis is characterized by mild swelling and injection of the conjunctiva.

2. **Treatment**

   a. **Topical decongestants:** Naphazoline 0.1% (Naphcon), phenylephrine (Neo-Synephrine), and oxymetazoline (OcuClear, Visine LR) may be used qid, alone or in combination with ophthalmic antihistamines such as antazoline (Vasocon-A) or pheniramine maleate (Naph-Con-A).

   b. Topical lodoxamide (Alomide) 0.1% ophthalmic solution, 1-2 drops qid, is helpful in more severe cases.

   c. Topical corticosteroids are helpful, but long-term use is not recommended; dexamethasone (Decadron) 1-2 drops tid-qid; TobraDex (tobramycin/dexamethasone 1-2 drops tid-qid.

V. Treatment of acute infectious conjunctivitis

A. Gonococcal ophthalmia neonatorum is treated with ceftriaxone (50 mg/kg/day IV/IM q24h) or cefotaxime (100 mg/kg/day IV/IM q12h) for 7 days.

B. Neonatal conjunctivitis caused by C trachomatis is treated with erythromycin, 50 mg/kg/day PO divided in 4 doses for 14 days.

C. Bacterial conjunctivitis among older infants and children is treated with polymyxin-bacitracin (Polysporin) ointment, applied to affected eye tid.

References, see page 182.

Cat and Dog Bites

Bite wounds account for approximately 1% of all emergency department visits: 10% of victims require suturing and 1-2% require hospitalization.

I. **Pathophysiology**
   A. **Dog bites** account for 80-90% of animal bites. Infection develops in 15-20% of dog bite wounds.
   B. **Cat bites** account for 15% of animal bites. Cat bites usually present as puncture wounds, of which 30-40% become infected.

II. **Clinical evaluation of bite wounds**
   A. **The circumstances of the injury** should be documented, and the animal's immunization status should be determined. It is important to determine whether the animal was provoked and to record the time of the injury.
   B. **The patient's tetanus immunization status**, current medications and allergies, history of chronic illness, immunocompromising conditions, immunosuppressive therapy, or a prosthetic valve or joint should be assessed.
   C. **The wound is measured** and classified as a laceration, puncture, crush injury or avulsion. Wounds are evaluated for evidence of injuries to tendons, joint spaces, blood vessels, nerves, and bone. A neurovascular examination and an assessment of wound depth should be completed.
   D. **Photographs** of the wound should be obtained if disfigurement has occurred or if litigation is anticipated.

III. **Laboratory and radiologic evaluation**
   A. **Radiographs** should be taken if there is considerable edema and tenderness around the wound or if bony penetration or foreign bodies are suspected.
   B. **Wounds seen within 8 to 24 hours after injury**, that have no signs of infection, do not require culture. If infection is present, aerobic and anaerobic cultures should be obtained.

IV. **Microbiology**
   A. **Bite wounds** usually have a polymicrobial contamination.
   B. **Pasteurella Multocida** is a gram-negative aerobe present in the oropharynx of dogs and cats. It is found in 20-30% of dog bite wounds and more than 50% of cat bite wounds.

Microorganisms Isolated from Infected Dog and Cat Bite Wounds	
Aerobes. Afipia felis, Capnocytophaga canimorsus, Eikenella corrodens, Enterobacter species, Flavobacterium species, Haemophilus aphrophilus, Moraxella species, Neisseria species, Pasteurella multocida, Pseudomonas species, Staphylococcus aureus, Staphylococcus epidermidis, Staphylococcus intermedius, Streptococci: alpha-hemolytic, beta-hemolytic, gamma-hemolytic	**Anaerobes.** Actinomyces, Bacteroides species, Eubacterium species, Fusobacterium species, Leptotrichia buccalis, Veillonella parvula
	Unusual Pathogens. Blastomyces dermatitidis, Francisella tularensis

V. **Management of dog and cat bites**
   A. **Wound care**
      1. The wound should be cleansed with 1% povidone iodine solution (Betadine), and irrigated with normal saline with a 20- to 50-mL syringe

with an Angiocath. Devitalized, crushed tissue should be sharply débrided.
2. Deep puncture wounds, wounds examined more than 24 hours after injury, clinically infected wounds, and bites of the hand should not be closed primarily.
3. Low-risk wounds seen within 24 hours after injury may be sutured; uninfected high-risk wounds seen 72 hours after initial injury may undergo delayed primary closure. Bites to the face and head have a good outcome and may be closed primarily.

B. **Antimicrobial therapy**
1. Prophylactic antibiotics are recommended for wounds that have a high risk of infection.
2. **High-risk bite wounds requiring prophylactic antibiotics**
   a. Full-thickness puncture wounds, severe crush injury and/or edema, wounds requiring debridement
   b. Cat bite wounds
   c. Bite wounds to the hand, foot or face; bone, joint, tendon or ligament, or wound adjacent to a prosthetic joint.
   d. Underlying diabetes, liver or pulmonary disease, history of splenectomy, malignancy, acquired immunodeficiency syndrome, or other immunocompromising condition.
3. Prophylactic antibiotic treatment is given for 3-7 days.

Prophylactic Antibiotics for Dog and Cat Bites	
Outpatient Antibiotics	
Penicillin V	**Adults:** 500 mg qid **Children:** 50 mg/kg/day, in divided doses q6-8h
Amoxicillin	**Adults:** 500 mg tid **Children:** 40 mg/kg/d, in divided doses tid
Cephalexin (Keflex)	**Adults:** 500 mg qid **Children:** 40 mg/kg/d PO qid
Doxycycline (Vibramycin)	**Adults:** 100 mg bid **Children:** 2-4 mg/kg/day, in divided doses bid
Amoxicillin/clavulanate (Augmentin)	**Adults:** 500 mg tid **Children:** 40 mg amoxicillin/kg/day, in divided doses tid
Ceftriaxone (Rocephin)	**Adults:** 1 g every 24 hours IM or IV **Children:** 50 mg/kg/d qd
Intravenous Antibiotic of choice	
Cefoxitin (Mefoxin)	**Adults:** 1-2 g q4-8h **Children:** 25-50 mg/kg/day, in divided doses q6h
Alternative Intravenous Antibiotics	
Ampicillin/sulbactam (Unasyn)	**Adults:** 1.5-3.0 g q6h

Ticarcillin-clavulanate (Timentin)	**Adults:** 3.1 g q6h
Ceftriaxone (Rocephin)	**Adults:** 1-2 g q24h **Children:** 50-100 mg/kg/day, in divided doses q24h

C. **Treatment of infected wounds.** Infected bite wounds are treated with amoxicillin/clavulanate (Augmentin). Cellulitis is treated for 10-14-days.

D. **Rabies immunoprophylaxis**
   1. The incidence of rabies in persons who have been bitten by a dog is very low because most dogs have been vaccinated. An untreated person has a less than 20% chance of contracting rabies from the bite of a rabid animal. However, if rabies is contracted, the mortality rate is 100%.
   2. Wild animals (raccoons, skunks, bats) are the most common source of rabies. Rabies is transmitted when the saliva of an infected animal comes into contact with the broken skin or mucosa of another mammal. The incubation period ranges from 10 days to one year.
   3. If rabies infection is suspected, rabies prophylaxis is administered as follows:
      a. **Rabies immune globulin (RIG),** 20 IU/kg, IM (separate from human diploid cell vaccine below).
      b. **Human diploid cell vaccine (HDCV),** 1 cc IM (not gluteal) given on days 1, 3, 7, 14, and 28.

E. **Tetanus Immunization.** Animal bites should be regarded as tetanus prone, although tetanus infection resulting from cat and dog bites is rare.

References, see page 182.

Cervical Adenopathy

Cervical lymph gland enlargement commonly occurs in children. In most cases the enlargement is a transient response to a benign local or generalized viral infection, and almost all children have small palpable cervical, axillary, and inguinal nodes. About 5% have small palpable suboccipital nodes. Distinctly uncommon are palpable postauricular, supraclavicular, epitrochlear, or popliteal nodes.

I. **Pathophysiology**
   A. The increase in size of a node may be the result of one of two processes: 1) proliferation of lymphocytes in the node or 2) infiltration by malignant cells or neutrophils.
   B. Often the cause of the adenopathy is obvious, such as with lymph glands draining an obvious source of infection. Malignancy is suggested by painless adenopathy in the posterior or lower cervical chains, particularly in older children. Almost all adenopathy in the anterior cervical triangle (anterior to the sternomastoid muscle) is benign. Fifty percent of masses in the posterior triangle are malignant.

II. **Etiology and epidemiology**
   A. **Infection** is the most common cause of cervical adenopathy in children.
   B. **Viral agents** are the most common infectious agents causing cervical adenopathy. Human herpesvirus 6, adenoviruses, herpes simplex virus, rubella, mumps virus, Epstein-Barr, cytomegalovirus, varicella, human

immunodeficiency virus and respiratory viruses may cause bilateral cervical adenitis.

C. **Bacterial infection** may be caused by oropharyngeal flora (anaerobes, group B streptococci, Staphylococcus aureus, Streptococcus pyogenes [GABS], atypical mycobacteria, Haemophilus sp, Actinomyces israelii, or Nocardia sp).

D. **Staphylococcus aureus and group A beta-hemolytic streptococci** account for 65-89% of acute unilateral infectious cervical adenitis in children. The majority occur in children ages 1 to 4 years.

E. **Group A beta-hemolytic Streptococci, Mycobacterium tuberculosis, or corynebacterium diphtheriae** may result form person-to-person spread by airborne droplets.

F. **Contact with domestic or wild animals or with feeding insects** may result in lymphadenitis due to Toxoplasma gondii, Francisella tularensis, Yersinia pestis, Rochalimaea henselae, or Pasteurella multocida.

G. **Cat-scratch disease (Bartonella henselae)** most often occurs after a lick or scratch from a cat or dog, or inoculation by a wood splinter, pin, fish hook, cactus spike, or porcupine quill.

Infectious Etiologies of Cervical Adenitis

Bacterial	Viral	Fungal/protozoal	Other
Localized Acute			
Staphylococcus aureus *Streptococcus pyogenes* Group B streptococcus Anaerobes *Francisella tularensis*	Rubella Adenoviruses Herpes simplex virus Mumps Human herpes-virus 6	Toxoplasmosis Histoplasmosis	Kawasaki syndrome Rickettsial pox
Subacute or Chronic			
Tuberculosis Atypical mycobacteria Cat-scratch disease	Syphilis Actinomycosis Nocardiosis		Brucellosis
Generalized			
Syphilis Tuberculosis Scarlet fever Typhoid fever Leptospirosis Brucellosis virus	HIV Epstein-Barr Cytomegalovirus Measles Rubella Varicella Adenovirus	Histoplasmosis Toxoplasmosis	Rickettsial Scrub typhus

H. **Toxoplasma gondii** may result from contact with cat feces, undercooked meat, or contaminated vegetables.

I. **Francisella tularensis** may be transmitted by direct contact with infected animals or their carcasses, by ingestion of water contaminated by animals, or by bites of ticks, deer flies, mosquitoes, or mites.

J. **Brucellosis** may result from contact with or ingestion of contaminated meat or dairy products, which can include those from cattle, swine, goats, dogs, or sheep.

K. **Leptospirosis** results most often from contact with water or soil contaminated by cats, dogs, rodents, or livestock.

L. **Pasteurella multocida** is an aerobic coccobacillus found in the normal flora of the mouth of many animals and occasionally of humans. Cellulitis and regional adenopathy most often occurs as the result of an animal bite.

M. **Atypical mycobacterial infections** occur typically in rural Caucasian children, 1 to 4 years of age, who have no history of exposure to tuberculosis. Involvement usually is unilateral and associated with a normal chest radiograph and a normal purified protein derivative (PPD) skin test.

N. **Mycobacterium tuberculosis** generally causes tubercular cervical adenitis in children who are urban and black, have a history of exposure to tuberculosis, have an abnormal chest radiograph, unilateral or bilateral involvement, and an abnormal PPD.

O. **Kawasaki syndrome** may cause unilateral cervical lymphadenopathy in infants and toddlers.

Organism Associated with Infectious Cervical Lymphadenitis
Neonates
Staphylococcus aureus Group B streptococcal "cellulitis-adenitis" syndrome
Infancy
As above Kawasaki syndrome
1 to 4 Years
Staphylococcus aureus Streptococcus pyogenes Atypical mycobacteria
5 to 15 years
Anaerobic bacteria Toxoplasmosis Cat-scratch disease Tuberculosis

III. **Clinical evaluation of cervical adenopathy**

A. **Seventy to 80% of acute unilateral cervical adenitis cases**, caused by GABS or staphylococcal infection, occur in those aged 1 to 4 years who frequently have a history of upper respiratory symptoms, including sore throat, earache, coryza, or impetigo. The submandibular nodes are involved most commonly.

B. **Group A beta-hemolytic streptococcal** disease should be suspected when impetigo or pharyngitis is present.

C. **Staphylococcus aureus and group B streptococci** are the most common causes of cervical lymphadenitis in newborn infants. In older infants whose mean age is 5 weeks, group B streptococcus causes the "cellulitis-adenitis" syndrome.

D. **A papular or pustular lesion** distal to the adenopathy, suggesting an inoculation site, should lead to consideration of tularemia, Nocardia, actinomycosis, plague, cutaneous diphtheria, and cat-scratch disease.

E. **Tularemia** is a disease of acute onset associated with fever, chills, and headaches. It is characterized by tender swollen lymph nodes and a painful swollen papule, which develops distal to the involved nodes. The papule then ruptures to form an ulcer. Fifty percent of the lymph nodes will suppurate and drain while the other 50% remain enlarged and tender for several months.

F. **Toxoplasmosis** most often is an asymptomatic infection accounting for 3-7% of significant adenopathy. The lymph nodes are discrete, rarely more than 3 cm in diameter, usually not tender, and do not suppurate. The clinical course is self-limited, lasting for up to 12 months.

G. **Cat-scratch disease** presents as a small papule that appears at the inoculation site 7 to 12 days after inoculation. Over the next 4 weeks, regional lymphadenitis appears. The involved regional lymph nodes are tender, warm, red, and indurated; up to 40% may suppurate. The lymphadenitis runs an indolent course of 4 to 6 weeks.

H. **Yersinia pestis** causes acute onset of fever, chills, headache, and weakness, which may be accompanied by a papule at the inoculation site. In bubonic plague, typical large, fixed, edematous and exquisitely tender nodes develop at one site.

I. **Brucellosis**, causes mild cervical or inguinal adenopathy, malaise, and fever within 1 week to several months of ingesting or inhaling the organism.

J. **Pasteurella multocida** infections cause an acute edematous cellulitis of the inoculation site, with fever, headache, and regional adenopathy.

IV. **Diagnosis of cervical adenopathy**

A. **Acute pyogenic bacterial infection** most often will be associated with an acute onset of 5 days or less, tender, enlarged nodes, and fever. The adenopathy may be bilateral if pharyngitis was the primary focus or unilateral if the focus is a dental or skin abscess. Associated generalized adenopathy suggests a generalized infection.

B. **Subacute or chronic adenopathy.** When the involved nodes are well localized, nontender, and unilateral, a granulomatous infection or malignancy is most likely.

1. A history of exposure to an individual who has tuberculosis or to ticks or other insects, cats, rodents, or other wild animals may suggest an etiology. If the adenopathy is generalized, tuberculosis, brucellosis, and histoplasmosis are more likely.

2. If the adenopathy is unilateral, an atypical mycobacterial infection or cat-scratch disease is more likely.

C. **Physical Examination.** Characteristics of the involved nodes and possible foci of infection or inoculate should be assessed. Fever, generalized adenopathy, hepatosplenomegaly, rash, joint swelling, and pulmonary findings should be sought.

D. **Tumors,** particularly neuroblastomas in younger children and lymphomas in older children, should be considered when evaluating any subacute or chronic, painless, firm, and noninflamed cervical mass. A malignancy is of particular concern in older children when the node is in the posterior triangle or extends across the sternomastoid muscle to involve the anterior triangle.

V. **Aspiration, biopsy, and laboratory tests**

A. **A specific diagnosis** of cervical adenitis depends either on demonstration of the organism by Gram stain, culture of aspirated or biopsied tissue, elevated IgM antibody titers, or skin testing. A complete blood count, erythrocyte sedimentation rate, liver function tests, or radiographic studies may help define the extent of involvement.

B. Needle aspiration of acutely inflamed nodes should be performed if 48 hours of antimicrobial therapy has failed, or if the infection is severe enough to require parenteral therapy.

C. Aspiration. After cleansing and anesthetizing the skin, the aspiration is performed with a 18- to 20-gauge needle and a 10- to 20-cc syringe. If no material is aspirated, 1 to 2 mL of sterile saline is injected and reaspirated.

D. Nodes should be incised and drained if pus is demonstrated on needle aspiration.

E. Excisional node biopsy should be performed for adenopathy suggestive of a malignancy. Excisional biopsy or incision and drainage are indicated for noninflamed hard nodes, nodes fixed to adjacent structures (particularly in the posterior triangle), and in older children, who have an increased incidence of lymphoma.

VI. Management of acute pyogenic bacterial lymphadenitis

Treatment of Acute Pyogenic Bacterial Lymphadenitis

Symptomatic Therapy

1. Apply warm, moist dressings
2. Prescribe analgesics
3. Incise and drain nodes that have suppuration

Antimicrobial Therapy

Suspected staphylococcal/group A and B streptococcal disease
  Cellulitis or marked enlargement, moderate-to-severe systemic symptoms, or in infants 1 mo of age:
    IV Nafcillin 150 mg/kg day or
    IV Cefazolin 150 mg/kg/day after aspiration of node
  Suppuration:
    IV antibiotics as above and incision and drainage
  No prominent systemic symptoms, cellulitis, or suppuration:
    Dicloxacillin 25 mg/kg/day or
    Cephalexin 50 mg/kg/day or
    Clindamycin 30 mg/kg/day
Suspected anaerobic infection with dental or periodontal disease, include:
    Penicillin V 50 mg/kg/day or
    Clindamycin 30 mg/kg/day or
Group A streptococcal infection
    Aqueous penicillin G 50 000 IU/kg/day IV or
    Penicillin V 50 mg/kg/day PO or
    Cephalexin 50 mg/kg/day PO or erythromycin ethylsuccinate 40 mg/kg/day PO
Group B streptococcal disease in infants
    Aqueous penicillin G 200 000 IU/kg/day IV, if sensitive.

References, see page 182.

Intestinal Helminths

Intestinal helminth infestations most commonly affect travelers, migrant laborers, refugees, children of foreign adoptions, and the homeless. These parasitic infections are associated with day care centers and overseas travel.

I. **Clinical evaluation**
   A. **Intestinal helminth infections are usually asymptomatic**, but serious infections may cause symptoms ranging from abdominal discomfort to severe pain. Anorexia nausea, diarrhea, pruritus, rectal prolapse, bowel obstruction, and death may occur. Hives and eosinophilia may develop, and the worms may sometimes spontaneously exit the body through the anus.
   B. **Stool examination.** Examination of the stool for ova and parasites is the most important test for helminthic infection. Stools are collected using plastic wrap under the toilet seat. Fresh stool may also be obtained by rectal examination.

II. **Enterobiasis**
   A. **The pinworm (Enterobius vermicularis)** is the most common helminth. Pinworms present as anal pruritus in irritable children. The disorder tends to occur in temperate climates. Many patients are asymptomatic. Heavier infections may cause insomnia, restlessness, vulvovaginitis, loss of appetite, and intractable anal itching.
   B. Pinworms are about 10 mm in length. The female worm has a pin-shaped tail. At night, worms migrate through the anus, then deposit their eggs and die on the perianal skin. Microscopic eggs infest clothing, bedding, and other surfaces, often spreading to the entire family.
   C. Pinworms are best diagnosed by examining the perianal skin. The stool is usually negative for ova and worms. To obtain the eggs, a tongue blade covered with clear tape is placed sticky-side down over the unwashed perianal skin in the morning. Specimens are collected on three separate mornings, then taped to glass slides and taken to a laboratory for examination.
   D. The elongate, colorless eggs measure 50 to 60 µm and are flattened on one side. Worms may also be visualized if the anus is examined late at night or early in the morning.
   E. **Treatment**
      1. **Mebendazole (Vermox)**, one 100-mg tablet orally, is safe and effective. A second dose is given 10 days later. The entire family is treated.
      2. Infested clothing and bedding are washed and fingernails should be kept trimmed, and the perianal area kept clean. Dogs and cats do not spread this infection. Relapses are common.

III. **Ascariasis**
   A. **Roundworms (Ascaris lumbricoides)** measure up to 18 inches in length. The infection is fairly common in the rural southeastern United States and is frequent among immigrants. A lumbricoides only infests humans.
   B. Ascaris eggs reach the soil in feces, and they may persist in the soil for more than a decade until they are accidentally consumed. In the gut, worms may cause intestinal obstruction. However, most patients experience only vague abdominal discomfort or nausea.
   C. **Treatment**
      1. Mebendazole (Vermox), 100 mg bid for three days.

2. A follow-up examination of stool for ova and parasites should be performed in two months. Family screening is recommended.

IV. Trichuriasis

A. Whipworm (Trichuris trichiura) infestation is less common than Ascaris infestation, occurring in the southeastern states and in foreign immigrants.

B. Whipworm eggs incubate in the soil. When swallowed, they travel to the colon.

C. Adult whipworms are 30-50 μm in length, with a thread-like anterior portion. They can live in the intestine and produce eggs for several years, causing mild blood loss and symptoms similar to proctitis and inflammatory bowel disease. Rectal prolapse, diarrhea, loss of appetite, and hives may occur.

D. Treatment of trichuriasis is the same as for ascariasis.

V. Less common parasites

A. Hookworms

1. Hookworms develop in the soil from eggs in feces. The larvae are capable of penetrating the bare feet and causing a pruritic rash. The larvae eventually reach the small intestine.

2. Adult hookworms are about 10 μm in length, with a hooked anterior end, which they use to consume 0.03-0.15 mL of blood per day for 10 to 15 years.

3. Manifestations include iron deficiency anemia, chronic fatigue, geophagia, failure to thrive, and depression.

4. Treatment consists of mebendazole and iron supplementation.

B. Strongyloidiasis

1. Filariform larvae are capable of penetrating intact skin, persisting for 40 years or more in the small intestine. It can also be spread in feces or as a sexually transmitted disease. Persistent unexplained eosinophilia in a patient from a region where Strongyloides infection is endemic should prompt serologic testing because stool specimens are often negative.

2. Symptoms of strongyloidiasis are usually absent but may include pruritus, pneumonia, abdominal cramping, and colitis. Treatment consists of thiabendazole (Mintezol).

C. Tapeworms

1. **Beef tapeworm** is transmitted by inadequately cooked beef, reaching up to 10 to 15 feet in length in the gut. Diagnosis is made by passage of ribbon-like tapeworm segments from the rectum or by finding the eggs in a stool.

2. **Pork tapeworm** is far more dangerous than T. saginata since its eggs can cause cysticercosis, the invasion of human tissue by developing larval forms. In severe cases, the larvae may invade the central nervous system, causing neurocysticercosis.

    a. Pork tapeworm is found in immigrants from Central and South America. Patients with neurocysticercosis frequently present with seizures.

    b. This diagnosis should be considered in the evaluation of a patient from Central or South America with a new-onset seizure disorder.

3. **Dwarf tapeworm** is the most common tapeworm in the U.S. This tapeworm is 1 inch in length. Ingestion of food contaminated with mouse droppings may spread the infection. H. nana infection may cycle in immigrant children for years.

4. **Fish tapeworm** is occasionally transmitted by undercooked fish, especially from the Great Lakes region. It can occasionally causes megaloblastic anemia.

5. **Treatment of all tapeworms** consists of praziquantel (Biltricide) or niclosamide (Niclocide).

References, see page 182.

Orbital and Periorbital Cellulitis

Periorbital cellulitis is a bacterial infection of the skin and structures superficial to the orbit; orbital cellulitis is a bacterial infection of the orbit.

I. **Pathogenesis of periorbital cellulitis**
   A. The most common causes of eyelid redness and swelling are allergy, trauma, and insect stings or bites.
   B. Periorbital cellulitis usually occurs after the skin near the eye has been broken by trauma, an insect bite, or infection with herpes simplex or varicella zoster viruses. The organisms that most frequently cause periorbital cellulitis following trauma are Staphylococcus aureus and Streptococcus pyogenes (group A beta-hemolytic streptococci).
   C. A bacterial pathogen is identified in only 30% of cases of periorbital cellulitis, and the pathogen is isolated from the blood in about two thirds of these cases.
   D. Since the introduction of H influenzae type b conjugate vaccines (HbCV), Hib disease accounts for fewer than 15% of periorbital cellulitis. A child who has received a second dose of HbCV more than 1 week before the onset of eyelid swelling is very unlikely to have HIB disease.

II. **Pathogenesis of orbital cellulitis**
   A. Orbital cellulitis may progress to subperiosteal abscess, orbital abscess, and cavernous sinus thrombosis.
   B. About one-fourth of isolates are S aureus; one-fifth, S pyogenes; one-fifth, HiB; one-tenth, S pneumoniae; one-tenth, anaerobic bacteria; and the remaining 15%, other bacteria.

III. **Clinical evaluation**
   A. Periorbital cellulitis usually occurs in children younger than 2 years of age. Clinical findings include a temperature of 39°C or more and a peripheral white blood cell count of greater than 15,000/mm³.
   B. Periorbital and orbital cellulitis cause eyelid swelling, with the swelling being unilateral in 95-98% of cases. Virtually all involved eyelids will be erythematous or violaceous (purple).
   C. Signs of trauma or local infection are observed in one-third of patients. Herpes simplex and varicella zoster virus infections of the eyelid can serve as a nidus for a secondary bacterial infection.
   D. When conjunctival inflammation, a purulent discharge, and bilateral lid involvement are present, the cause is much more likely to be conjunctivitis, rather than periorbital or orbital cellulitis.
   E. **Globe displacement (proptosis), abnormal movement (ophthalmoplegia), or pain on movement** should be sought, and visual acuity should be tested.
   F. **Laboratory evaluation**
      1. **White blood cell count** greater than 15,000/mm³ suggests bacteremic disease.
      2. **Lumbar puncture** should be performed on all children younger than 1 year of age who have periorbital or orbital cellulitis and who have not had at least two doses of H influenzae B vaccine.
      3. **Blood culture for bacterial pathogens** should be obtained from all

children who have periorbital or orbital cellulitis. Specimens of purulent material from wounds near the affected eye also should be cultured.

IV. Treatment

A. Orbital cellulitis.
Children who have signs of orbital cellulitis should be hospitalized, and antimicrobial therapy should provide coverage for the pathogens most commonly associated with sinusitis as well as for S aureus and anaerobes. A third-generation cephalosporin, such as ceftriaxone (50 mg/kg qd IM or IV) or cefotaxime (50 mg/kg/dose q6h IV), plus clindamycin (10 mg/kg/dose q8h IV) will provide excellent coverage.

B. Periorbital cellulitis
1. Periorbital cellulitis can be managed on an outpatient basis if there is no orbital involvement and the child does not appear toxic. If a purulent wound is present near the involved eyelid, the child should be hospitalized.
2. Ceftriaxone (50 mg/kg, not to exceed 1 g) is given IM or IV. If the blood culture remains negative, the child may be started on a broad-spectrum oral agent such as ampicillin/clavulanate (Augmentin) or trimethoprim/sulfamethoxazole (Bactrim) to complete a 7- to 10-day course of therapy.
3. **Purulent wounds** near the involved eyelid are likely to have S aureus or S pyogenes infection and require treatment with a parenteral beta-lactamase-resistant agent, such as oxacillin or nafcillin, a first-generation cephalosporin [cefazolin (Ancef) 50-100 mg/kg/d q6-8h or cephalothin (Keflin) 75 mg/kg/day IM/IV q6h], or a macrolide (clindamycin 40 mg/kg/day IV q8h).

References, see page 182.

Tuberculosis

The number of cases of tuberculosis in children younger than five years of age in cities has increased 94.3% in the last four years.

I. Natural history of tuberculosis

A. Tuberculosis infection is initiated by the inhalation of organisms into the lung. During an incubation period that lasts 2 to 10 weeks, the organisms spread to the hilar lymph nodes. The condition is now considered primary tuberculosis. During the incubation period, the purified protein derivative (PPD) test usually becomes positive.

B. **Primary tuberculosis** is often completely asymptomatic, and the chest radiograph may be only minimally abnormal, with hilar adenopathy, and/or small parenchymal infiltrates. Healed primary tuberculosis may leave calcified deposits in the lung parenchyma and/or hilum.

C. **Extrapulmonary disease** is more common in children than in adults. In children, 25% of tuberculosis disease is extrapulmonary. Children and young adolescents are more likely than adults to have tuberculous meningitis, miliary tuberculosis, adenitis, and bone and joint infections.

D. Pulmonary disease develops in 40% of children younger than one year of age who have untreated tuberculosis. Untreated children between one and five years of age have a 24% risk of pulmonary tuberculosis, and untreated adolescents 11 to 15 years of age have a 15% risk.

E. Children who do not have clinical disease, but who harbor a reservoir of quiescent organisms may develop tuberculous disease later in life. Reactivation is most likely to occur during adolescence, during an episode of immunosuppression, in the presence of chronic disease, or in the elderly.

II. Diagnosis of tuberculosis in children

A. Children exposed to tuberculosis

1. All household contacts of adults with active disease should be tested by PPD. Thirty to 50% of all household contacts of infectious adults will have a positive PPD.

2. Children who are known contacts and who are PPD negative, should receive prophylactic therapy, usually isoniazid (Laniazid), 10 mg/kg/day. The PPD is repeated in 3 months to check for conversion to a positive PPD test, which would indicate infection. If the repeat PPD test remains negative, the child is assumed not to be infected, and prophylactic therapy can be discontinued. If the repeat PPD test is positive, the child should be treated for 9 months.

3. Any child with a positive PPD test should be evaluated for active pulmonary and extrapulmonary tuberculosis with a history and physical examination and posteroanterior and lateral chest radiographs. The source of the child's infection should be determined, and the susceptibility of the source case's M. tuberculosis strain is considered in selecting a prophylactic or treatment regimen. Contact with the person with contagious tuberculosis who infected the child must be prevented until the source case is no longer infectious.

B. Children at risk for infection

1. A PPD test is recommended for children in high-risk groups. A screening PPD test of 5 tuberculin units can be placed before a dose of measles-mumps-rubella (MMR) vaccine, simultaneously with the MMR vaccine dose, or 6 weeks after the MMR vaccine dose. A false-negative PPD test may occur within 6 weeks of an MMR vaccination, because of transient immunosuppression from the live MMR vaccine.

2. The size of the PPD reaction determined to be positive varies with the risk of tuberculous infection. The diameter of the induration is measured 48 to 72 hours after PPD placement. A positive PPD test requires an evaluation for tuberculous disease.

Criteria for a Positive PPD Test in Children

Reaction of 5 mm or more

Children suspected of having tuberculosis (chest x-ray consistent with active or previously active tuberculosis; clinical signs of tuberculosis)

Children in close contact with persons who have known or suspected infectious tuberculosis

Children with immunosuppressive conditions (HIV infection, corticosteroid therapy)

Reaction of 10 mm or more
Children younger than 4 years of age
Children born in, or whose parents were born in, regions where tuberculosis is highly prevalent
Children frequently exposed to adults who are HIV infected, homeless persons, IV and other street drug users, poor and medically indigent city dwellers, residents of nursing homes, incarcerated or institutionalized persons, and migrant farm workers
Children with other medical risk factors (Hodgkin's disease, lymphoma, diabetes mellitus, chronic renal failure)

Reaction of 15 mm or more
Children older than 4 years without any risk factors

3. Previous vaccination with bacille Calmette-Guerin (BCG) vaccine does not change the interpretation of the PPD test because there is no way to distinguish infection from a reaction to BCG vaccine.
4. High tuberculous infection rates occur in Southeast Asia, Africa, Eastern Mediterranean countries, Western Pacific countries, Mexico, the Caribbean, and South and Central America.
C. **Clinical evidence suggestive of tuberculosis.** Tuberculosis must be considered when a child presents with pneumonia that is unresponsive to antibiotic treatment, "aseptic" meningitis, joint or bone infection, hilar or cervical adenopathy, or pleural effusion.

III. **Evaluation of tuberculosis in children**
   A. The work-up for a child with a positive PPD test or suspected tuberculosis includes the following:
      1. **History.** Risk factors for exposure to tuberculosis; symptoms of tuberculosis; adult source case.
      2. **Physical examination.** Adenopathy, positive respiratory system findings, bone or joint disease, meningitis.
      3. **Diagnostic tests**
         a. Chest x-ray (posteroanterior and lateral).
         b. Gastric aspirates in children who are too young to produce a deep sputum sample
         c. Sputum collection or induction in children who are able to produce a deep sputum sample.
         d. Cultures and smears of appropriate body fluids in children with suspected extrapulmonary tuberculosis.

IV. **Treatment of active tuberculosis**
   A. Treatments should be directly observed to ensure compliance. If possible, the susceptibility results of the adult source case should guide the medication choice. If the organism may be resistant to one of the standard medications, ethambutol (Myambutol) (or streptomycin in children too young for visual acuity testing) should be included.
   B. Drug-resistant tuberculosis should be suspected in children who are exposed to immigrants from Asia, Africa and Latin America, children who live in large cities, or who are from areas in which isoniazid resistance occurs in more than 4% of cases, children who are homeless, children who have previously been treated for tuberculosis, and children who are exposed to adults at high risk for tuberculosis.

Treatment Regimens for Tuberculosis		
Type of Disease	**Primary Regimen**	**Comments**
Pulmonary disease	Two months of isoniazid, 10-15 mg/kg/day, max 300 mg/day; rifampin (Rifadin), 10-20 mg/kg/day, max 600 mg/day; and pyrazinamide, 20-40 mg/kg/day, max 2.0 g/day, followed by 4 months of daily or twice-weekly isoniazid and rifampin	Medications can be given 2 or 3 times/week under direct observation in the initial phase
Extrapulmonary disease, except meningitis, miliary disease and bone/joint disease	Same as for pulmonary disease	
Meningitis, miliary disease, and bone/joint disease	Two months of daily isoniazid, rifampin, pyrazinamide and streptomycin, followed by 10 months of daily or twice-weekly isoniazid and rifampin	

V. **Prophylactic treatment of tuberculosis infection**
   A. Children with a positive PPD test, but no signs of disease should receive isoniazid for 9 months if they are younger than 18 years and for at least 6 months if they are 18 years of age or older. Exposure to drug-resistant tuberculosis requires more specific therapy.
   B. The child with tuberculous infection or disease may return to school or child care after drug therapy has been initiated and clinical symptoms have resolved. HIV testing should be completed for any older child or adult with tuberculosis.

References, see page 182.

Urinary Tract Infection

Urinary tract infection (UTI) is common in infants and children, and, if untreated, it can cause irreversible chronic renal failure.

I. **Epidemiology**
   A. One to 2% of newborn girls and boys have UTIs. In infancy and childhood, UTI is more common in girls than in boys; 1% of school-age girls develop symptomatic infection each year.
   B. Risk factors for UTI in females include sexual intercourse, sexual abuse, use of bubble bath, constipation, pinworms, and infrequent or incomplete voiding. In either sex, risk factors include ureteric reflux in a sibling, urologic abnormalities, indwelling urethral catheterization, and neurogenic bladder.
II. **Pathophysiology**
   A. UTI usually is caused by bacteria that ascend up the urethra into the bladder. E coli is the most common organism associated with UTI.

B. Other enteric bacteria include Klebsiella, Enterococcus sp, and Staphylococcus saprophyticus (a common cause in males which can also occur in females).

III. Clinical evaluation

A. In prepubertal children, UTI usually does not cause frequency, dysuria, or urgency.

B. In the newborn, signs of UTI may include late-onset jaundice, hypothermia, signs of sepsis, failure to thrive, vomiting, and fever. In infants and preschool children, additional findings include diarrhea and strong-smelling urine.

C. The school-age child may complain of frequency, dysuria, and urgency, but enuresis, strong-smelling urine, and vomiting also are common.

Signs and Symptoms of UTI In Children		
Newborns	**Infants and Preschoolers**	**School Age Children**
Jaundice	Diarrhea	Vomiting
Hypothermia	Failure to thrive	Fever
Sepsis	Vomiting	Strong-smelling urine
Failure to thrive	Fever	Abdominal pain
Vomiting	Strong-smelling urine	Frequency
Fever		Dysuria
		Urgency
		Enuresis

D. Physical examination

1. The growth curve should be reviewed because children who have frequent UTIs may have a decreased rate of growth. Failure to thrive is not uncommon among infants and newborns who have UTI.

2. Chronic renal failure secondary to UTIs may cause hypertension. The abdominal examination may reveal tenderness or a mass may indicate an enlarged bladder or obstructed urinary tract.

3. Signs of vaginitis, labial adhesions, local irritation, or sexual activity/abuse should be sought. The urinary stream should be evaluated in males.

4. A tight phimosis in an uncircumcised male infant may predispose to UTI. A rectal examination may detect masses or poor sphincter tone, indicative of a neurogenic bladder.

IV. Laboratory evaluation

A. For children who have moderate-to-severe symptoms (eg, fever, vomiting, failure to thrive, signs of sepsis), the urine specimen should be collected by catheter or suprapubic aspiration.

1. Bag urine specimens are always contaminated and are not recommended for symptomatic patients. Bag urine specimens are useful only when negative.

2. Urinalysis. Urine is examined by dipstick and microscopic analysis. The nitrate test is more specific for UTI than leukocyte esterase. Centrifuged urine is examined for white blood cells or bacteria.

3. Pyuria. >10 WBC/mm^3 detected by microscopic analysis of an uncentrifuged specimen combined with a Gram stain analysis showing the presence of bacteria is associated with a positive urine culture in 90%.

B. In children who have mild symptoms, a clean-catch urine specimen should be tested by dipstick urinalysis. If the nitrite test is negative, urine microscopy is performed; if microscopy is negative, the specimen should be cultured.

Culture Criteria for Significant Bacteriuria	
Method	**Colony Count**
Suprapubic aspiration	Any bacteria
Urethral catheterization	>10,000 cfu/mL
Best catch	$\geq$50,000 cfu/mL

V. Management

A. Patients who have severe symptoms should be treated initially with two parenteral antibiotics that provide coverage for both gram-positive and gram-negative organisms.

B. For children whose infections are mild, a single oral antibiotic to which the patient has not been exposed recently is prescribed.

Antibiotic Therapy for Urinary Tract Infections with Severe Symptoms	
Agent	**Dosage (mg /kg/day)**
Neonate	
Ampicillin and Gentamicin	7.5 mg/kg/day IV/IM q8h 100 mg/kg/day IV/IM q6h
Older Child	
Ceftriaxone (Rocephin)	50 mg /kg/day (IM, IV) q24h
Cefotaxime (Claforan)	100 mg /kg/day (IV) q6-8h
Ampicillin/sulbactam (Unasyn)	100-200 mg of ampicillin/kg/day q6h
Gentamicin	3-7.5 mg /kg/day(IV, IM) q8h

Antibiotic Therapy for Urinary Tract Infections with Mild Symptoms	
Agent	**Dosage**
Cefpodoxime (Vantin)	10 mg/kg/day PO q12h [susp: 50 mg/5 mL, 100 mg/5 mL; tabs: 100 mg, 200 mg]
Cefprozil (Cefzil)	30 mg/kg/day PO q12h [susp: 125 mg/5 mL, 250 mg/5 mL; tabs: 250, 500 mg]

Agent	Dosage
Cefixime (Suprax)	8 mg/kg/d PO qd-bid [susp: 100 mg/5 mL, tab: 200,400 mg]
Cefuroxime (Ceftin)	125-500 mg PO q12h [125, 250, 500 mg]
Amoxicillin/clavulanate (Augmentin)	40 mg of amoxicillin kg/day PO q8h [susp: amoxicillin 125 mg/clavulanate/5 mL; tab: amoxicillin 250 mg/clavulanate; amoxicillin 500 mg/clavulanate]
Trimethoprim/sulfamethoxazole (Bactrim)	6-12 mg/kg/day (trimethoprim) q12h [susp: trimethoprim 40 mg/sulfamethoxazole 200 mg/5 mL]

- C. A urine culture should be repeated early in the course of treatment if symptoms persist.
- D. Most patients are treated for 10 days; those treated parenterally can be switched to oral therapy when symptoms have resolved and antimicrobial susceptibilities are known.
- E. **Follow-up screening.** After the first infection is treated successfully, follow-up screening for UTI is indicated at 1 month, 3 months, 6 months, 12 months, and yearly. Home nitrite testing on first-morning urine specimens is an accurate method for follow-up.

VI. Imaging studies
- A. Imaging studies are recommended in the following patients:
    1. UTI in a male.
    2. UTI in an infant.
    3. Pyelonephritis in a female.
    4. Recurrent UTI in a female.
- B. Early renal ultrasonography should be obtained to look for evidence of urinary tract obstruction. If results show abnormalities, radioactive renal scanning is useful for defining renal anatomy more precisely.
- C. A voiding cystourethrogram should be performed 3 to 6 weeks after symptoms have resolved in order to define urethral and bladder anatomy. Children who have UTI with simple reflux usually can be observed as long as recurrent infection is prevented.

VII. Prevention of recurrent urinary tract infection
- A. Uncircumcised males with phimosis may benefit from circumcision. Front-to-back wiping should be encouraged, bubble baths should be eliminated, showers encouraged, and pinworms should be treated.
- B. A high fluid intake and a frequent voiding schedule is recommended. Constipation should be identified and treated. Patients with postcoital UTI should void after intercourse and perhaps take antimicrobial prophylaxis after intercourse.
- C. Patients with significant ureteral reflux ≥grade 1, and those with frequent recurrences require long-term (6 months to 2 years) prophylaxis, which can be achieved with sulfisoxazole (Gantrisin), 30 mg/kg qhs.

References, see page 182.

Viral Laryngotracheitis (Croup)

Acute laryngotracheitis (viral croup) is the most common infectious cause of acute upper airway obstruction in pediatrics, causing 90% of cases. The disease is usually self-limited. Children in the 1-2-year-old age group are most commonly affected. Viral croup affects 3-5% of all children each year. Croup is most common from the late fall to early spring, although cases may occur throughout the year.

I. **Clinical evaluation of upper airway obstruction and stridor**
   A. **Stridor** is the most common presenting feature of all causes of acute upper airway obstruction. It is a harsh sound that results from air movement through a partially obstructed upper airway.
      1. **Supraglottic disorders**, such as epiglottitis, cause quiet, wet stridor, a muffled voice, dysphagia and a preference for sitting upright.
      2. **Subglottic lesions**, such as croup, cause loud stridor accompanied by a hoarse voice and barky cough.
   B. **Patient age**
      1. Upper airway obstruction in school age and older children tends to be caused by severe tonsillitis or peritonsillar abscesses.
      2. From infancy to 2 years of age, viral croup and retropharyngeal abscess are the most common causes of upper airway obstruction.
   C. **Mode of onset**
      1. Gradual onset of symptoms, usually preceded by upper respiratory infection symptoms, suggests viral croup, severe tonsillitis or retropharyngeal abscess.
      2. Very acute onset of symptoms suggests epiglottitis.
      3. A history of a choking episode or intermittent respiratory distress suggests a foreign body inhalation.
      4. Facial edema and urticaria suggests angioedema.
   D. **Emergency management of upper airway obstruction**
      1. Maintaining an adequate airway takes precedence over other diagnostic interventions. If a supraglottic disorder is suspected, a person skilled at intubation must accompany the child at all times.
      2. Patients with suspected epiglottitis, severe respiratory distress from an obstruction, or suspected foreign body inhalation should be taken to the operating room for direct laryngoscopic visualization and possible intubation.

Causes of Upper Airway Obstruction in Children

Supraglottic Infectious Disorders
  Epiglottitis
  Peritonsillar abscess
  Retropharyngeal abscess
  Severe tonsillitis

Subglottic Infectious Disorders
  Croup (viral laryngotracheitis)
  Spasmodic croup
  Bacterial tracheitis

Non-Infectious Causes
  Angioedema
  Foreign body aspiration
  Congenital obstruction
  Neoplasms
  External trauma to neck

Causes of Upper Airway Obstruction in Children

	Epiglottitis	Laryngotra- cheobronchitis (Croup)	Bacterial Tracheitis	Foreign Body Aspiration
History				
Incidence in children presenting with stridor	8%	88%	2%	2%
Onset	Rapid, 4-12 hours	Prodrome, 1-7 days	Prodrome, 3 days, then 10 hours	Acute or chronic
Age	1-6 years	3 mo-3 years	3 mo-2 years	Any
Season	None	October-May	None	None
Etiology	Haemophilus influenza	Parainfluenza viruses	Staphylococ- cus	Many
Pathology	Inflammatory edema of epi- glottis and supraglottitis	Edema and inflammation of trachea and bronchial tree	Tracheal- bronchial edema, nec- rotic debris	Localized tracheitis
Signs and Symptoms				
Dysphagia	Yes	No	No	Rare
Difficulty swallowing	Yes	No	Rare	No
Drooling	Yes	No	Rare	No

	Epiglottitis	Laryngotra-cheobronchitis (Croup)	Bacterial Tracheitis	Foreign Body Aspiration
Stridor	Inspiratory	Inspiratory and expiratory	Inspiratory	Variable
Voice	Muffled	Hoarse	Normal	Variable
Cough	No	Barking	Variable	Yes
Temperature	Markedly elevated	Minimally elevated	Moderate	Normal
Heart rate	Increased early	Increased late	Proportional to fever	Normal
Position	Erect, anxious, "air hungry," supine position exacerbates	No effect on airway obstruction	No effect	No effect
Respiratory rate	Increased early	Increased late	Normal	Increased if bronchial obstruction present

Differentiation of Epiglottitis from Viral Laryngotracheitis		
Clinical Feature	Epiglottitis	Viral Croup
Retractions	present	present
Wheezing	absent	occasionally present
Cyanosis	present	present in severe cases
"Toxicity"	present	absent
Preference for sitting	yes	no

II. **Epidemiology and etiology of viral laryngotracheitis (Croup)**
   A. **Parainfluenza virus type 1** causes 40% of all cases of laryngotracheitis. Parainfluenza type 3, respiratory syncytial virus (RSV), parainfluenza type 2, and rhinovirus may also cause croup.
   B. RSV commonly affects infants younger than 12 months of age, causing wheezing and stridor. Influenza viruses A and B and mycoplasma have been implicated in patients older than 5 years.

III. **Clinical manifestations**
   A. Viral croup begins gradually with a 1-2 day prodrome, resembling an upper respiratory infection. Subglottic edema and inflammation of the larynx, trachea, and bronchi eventually develop.
   B. Low-grade fever and nocturnal exacerbation of cough are common. As airway obstruction increases retractions, develop, restlessness, anxiety, tachycardia, and tachypnea may occur.
   C. Cyanosis is a late sign. Severe obstruction leads to respiratory muscle exhaustion, hypoxemia, carbon dioxide accumulation, and respiratory

acidosis. Stridor becomes less apparent as muscle fatigue worsens.

    D. Ten percent of croup patients have severe respiratory compromise requiring hospital admission, and 3% of those children need airway support.

IV. **Laboratory evaluation**. The diagnosis of viral croup is based primarily on the history and clinical findings. When the diagnosis is uncertain or the patient requires hospitalization, x-rays can be helpful. The posteroanterior neck radiograph of a patient with viral croup shows symmetrical narrowing of the subglottic space ("steeple sign").

V. **Inpatient treatment of laryngotracheitis**

    A. The majority of patients who have croup do not require hospitalization.

    B. **Indications for hospitalization**

        1. Dusky or cyanotic skin color.

        2. Decreased air entry on auscultation.

        3. Severe stridor.

        4. Significant retractions.

        5. Agitation, restlessness, or obtundation.

    C. Signs that indicate the need for an artificial airway include decreased respiratory effort and decreased level of consciousness. Pulse oximetry may aid in assessing the severity of respiratory compromise.

    D. All patients suspected of having viral croup should be given humidified air. Hypoxic or cyanotic patients require oxygen via mask and may require intubation. Oral hydration is essential to help loosen secretions; however, intravenous hydration may become necessary in the very ill child.

    E. **Racemic epinephrine** has alpha-adrenergic properties, which decrease subglottic inflammation and edema.

        1. Racemic epinephrine is administered as 0.5 mL of a 2.25% solution, diluted with 3.5 mL of saline (1:8) by nebulization. It is given every 20-30 minutes for severe croup, and it is given every 4-6 hours for moderate croup.

    F. **Corticosteroids** reduce subglottic edema and inflammation.

        1. **Dexamethasone** (0.6 mg/kg IM) given one time early in the course of croup results in a shorter hospital stay and reduces cough and dyspnea.

        2. The need for intubation is reduced from 1.2% to 0.1%. Patients who do not require hospitalization should not receive steroids.

    G. **Acetaminophen** decreases fever and oxygen consumption in the febrile patient with croup.

VI. **Outpatient treatment of laryngotracheitis**

    A. Patients with mild viral croup usually are not admitted to the hospital and can be treated safely at home. Vaporizers, oral fluids, and antipyretics are the mainstays of home therapy.

    B. The prognosis for croup is good; however, a subset of children who have croup will later be identified as having asthma.

References, see page 182.

Pelvic Inflammatory Disease

Pelvic inflammatory disease (PID) is a polymicrobial genital tract infection that occurs in sexually active females. *Neisseria gonorrhoeae* and *Chlamydia trachomatis* are usually the causative agents of PID. Consequences of PID include chronic pain, ectopic pregnancy, and infertility. Sexually active females have a tenfold increase in risk compared with adults.

I. **Clinical evaluation**
   A. The most common presenting complaint of PID is lower abdominal pain. Associated symptoms include vaginal discharge, irregular bleeding, dysmenorrhea, dyspareunia, dysuria, nausea, vomiting, and fever. Most women who have acute PID present during the first half of the menstrual cycle.
   B. Empiric treatment should be undertaken if lower abdominal tenderness, adnexal tenderness, and cervical motion tenderness are present on physical examination.

II. **Laboratory diagnosis**
   A. A urine pregnancy test should be obtained to exclude the possibility of uterine or ectopic pregnancy. If an abnormal vaginal discharge is present, a sample should be examined microscopically for trichomoniasis, candidiasis, and bacterial vaginosis. Most patients should be evaluated with urinalysis and urine culture for urinary tract infection and a serologic test for syphilis. All patients who have STDs should be offered HIV testing.
   B. Endocervical samples should be examined for *C trachomatis* and *N gonorrhoeae*.
   C. *Chlamydia trachomatis* cell culture detects fewer than 80% of chlamydial infections. Antigen detection tests, which include direct-smear fluorescent antibody (DFA) and enzyme-linked immunosorbent assay (ELISA), are less sensitive and specific. Nucleic acid hybridization or genetic probe tests detect 50% to 70% of infections. Genetic amplification, which includes polymerase chain reaction (PCR) and ligase chain reaction (LCR), have detection rates of 95%, and the tests can be performed on vaginal and urine samples as well as on cervical samples.
   D. Although endocervical culture has been used traditionally for the detection of *N gonorrhoeae*, LCR now offers a readily available alternative. Its sensitivity and specificity for *N gonorrhoeae* exceeds 97%, and the same specimen can be used to test for both *N gonorrhoeae* and *C trachomatis*.
   E. Pelvic ultrasonography should be performed in patients with a positive pregnancy test. Beyond 6 weeks' gestation, the absence of an intrauterine sac on ultrasonography raises suspicion of an ectopic pregnancy. Laparoscopy rarely is necessary to establish the diagnosis of PID. It is indicated only when the diagnosis is in doubt or the patient has failed to respond to antibiotic therapy.

III. **Management**

CDC Recommendations for the Parenteral Treatment of Pelvic Inflammatory Disease
Parenteral Regimen A
Cefotetan (Cefotan) 2 g IV every 12 hours *OR* Cefoxitin (Mefoxin) 2 g IV every 6 hours *PLUS* Doxycycline 100 mg IV or orally every 12 hours

Parenteral Regimen B

Clindamycin 900 mg IV every 8 hours
PLUS
Gentamicin loading dose IV or IM (2 mg/kg of body weight), followed by a maintenance dose (1.5 mg/kg) every 8 hours. Single daily dosing may be substituted.

Alternative Parenteral Regimens

Ofloxacin (Floxin) 400 mg IV every 12 hours
PLUS
Metronidazole 500 mg IV every 8 hours
OR
Ampicillin/Sulbactam (Augmentin) 3 g IV every 6 hours
PLUS
Doxycycline 100 mg IV or orally every 12 hours
OR
Ciprofloxacin (Cipro) 200 mg IV every 12 hours
PLUS
Doxycycline 100 mg IV or orally every 12 hours
PLUS
Metronidazole 500 mg IV every 8 hours

CDC Recommendations for the Oral Treatment of Pelvic Inflammatory Disease

Oral Regimen A

Ofloxacin (Floxin) 400 mg orally twice a day for 14 days
PLUS
Metronidazole 500 mg orally twice a day for 14 days

Oral Regimen B

Ceftriaxone (Rocephin) 250 mg IM once
OR
Cefoxitin (Mefoxin) 2 g IM plus probenecid 1 g orally in a single dose concurrently once
OR
Other parenteral third-generation cephalosporin (eg, ceftizoxime or cefotaxime)
PLUS
Doxycycline 100 mg orally twice a day for 14 days

A. Patients who have baseline laboratory documentation of *N gonorrhoeae* or *C trachomatis* should be screened again following completion of therapy. Sexual partners of women who have PID should be treated for *N gonorrhoeae* and *C trachomatis*.

References, see page 182.

Gastrointestinal Disorders

Acute Abdominal Pain

The evaluation of abdominal pain is problematic because the pain is often difficult to localize, and the history in children is often nonspecific.

I. **Localization of abdominal pain**
   A. **Generalized pain** in the epigastrium usually comes from the stomach, duodenum, or the pancreas.
   B. **Periumbilical pain** usually originates in small bowel and colon or spleen.
   C. **Parietal pain,** caused by inflammation, is usually well localized.
   D. **Referred abdominal pain** occurs when poorly localized visceral pain is felt at a distant location.
      1. **Pancreatitis, cholecystitis, liver abscess,** or a splenic hemorrhage cause diaphragmatic irritation, which is referred to the ipsilateral neck and shoulders.
      2. **Intraabdominal fluid** may produce shoulder pain on reclining.
      3. **Gallbladder pain** may be felt in the lower back or infrascapular area.
      4. **Pancreatic pain** often is referred to the posterior flank.
      5. **Ureterolithiasis** often presents as pain radiating toward the ipsilateral groin.
      6. **Rectal or gynecological pain** often is perceived as sacral pain.
      7. **Right lower lobe pneumonia** may be perceived as right upper quadrant abdominal pain.
II. **Clinical evaluation**
   A. **History** should include the quality, timing, and type of abdominal pain.
      1. **Pain of sudden onset** often denotes colic, perforation or acute ischemia caused by torsion or volvulus.
      2. **Slower onset** of pain suggests inflammatory conditions, such as appendicitis, pancreatitis, or cholecystitis.
   B. **Colic** results from spasms of a hollow viscus organ secondary to an obstruction. It is characterized by severe, intermittent cramping, followed by intervals when the pain is present but less intense. Colic pain usually originates from the biliary tree, pancreatic duct, gastrointestinal tract, urinary system, or uterus and tubes.
   C. **Inflammatory pain** is caused by peritoneal irritation, and the patient presents quietly without much motion and appears ill. The pain is initially less severe and is exacerbated by movement.
   D. **Vomiting.** Usually abdominal pain will precede vomiting. The interval between abdominal pain and vomiting is shorter when associated with colic Delayed vomiting for many hours is often associated with distal bowel obstruction or ileus secondary to peritonitis.
   E. **Diarrhea.** Mild diarrhea with the onset of abdominal pain suggests acute gastroenteritis or early appendicitis. Delayed onset of diarrhea may indicate a perforated appendicitis, with the inflamed mass causing irritation of the sigmoid colon.
   F. **Physical examination**
      1. The abdomen should be observed, auscultated, and palpated for distention, localized tenderness, masses, and peritonitis. The groin must be examined

to exclude an incarcerated hernia or ovary, or torsion of an ovary or testicle.
2. **Rectal examination**
   a. **Gross blood in the stool** suggests ectopic gastric mucosa, Meckel's diverticula, or polyps.
   b. **Blood and mucus** (currant jelly stool) suggests inflammatory bowel disease or intussusception.
   c. **Melena** suggests upper gastrointestinal bleeding, necessitating gastric aspiration for blood.
   d. **Tests for occult blood** in the stool should be performed.
3. **Pelvic examinations** are mandatory for postmenarchal and/or sexually active female patients. The rectal examination may also be used to evaluate the cervix, uterus, adnexa, and other pelvic masses.
4. **Fever**
   a. Thoracic disease (eg, pneumonia) may be the cause of abdominal pain associated with fever.
   b. Costovertebral angle tenderness with fever suggests pyelonephritis or a high retrocecal appendicitis.

III. **Appendicitis**
   A. **Fever, vomiting, irritability, lethargy with right lower quadrant (RLQ) tenderness and guarding** are diagnostic of appendicitis in the very young patient until proven otherwise. A mass may be felt on rectal exam in 2-7% of younger patients with appendicitis.
   B. **Children older than 2 years old** present with a perforated appendix about 30-60% of the time. This incidence declines as the age of the child increases.
   C. **Lower abdominal pain in the adolescent female** may be caused by pelvic inflammatory disease (PID), ovarian cysts, ovarian torsion, ectopic pregnancy, or mittelschmerz (pain with ovulation).
   D. A WBC >15,000 supports the need for surgery, but a normal WBC and differential does not exclude appendicitis. An ultrasound of the appendix may reveal the diagnosis.

IV. **Intussusception**
   A. Intussusception is the most common cause of bowel obstruction between 2 months and 5 years of age. The most vulnerable age group is 4-10 months old, but children up to 7 years old may be at risk.
   B. Intussusception is characterized by vomiting, colicky abdominal pain (85%) with drawing up of the legs, and currant jelly stools (60%). Fever is common. Lethargy, dehydration, obtundation and/or coma may occur in younger infants.
   C. The abdomen may be soft and nontender between episodes of colicky pain, but eventually it becomes distended. A sausage-shaped mass in the right upper quadrant (RUQ) may be palpable.
   D. Intussusception may sometimes be palpated during rectal examination, and three percent of intussusceptions may prolapse. Ninety-five percent of intussusceptions are located at the ileocecal junction, and 5% are found elsewhere in the GI tract.
   E. **Abdominal x-ray.** The leading edge of the intussusception is usually outlined with air, which will establish the diagnosis. Often there are radiographic signs of bowel obstruction. When the plain abdominal x-ray is normal, intussusception cannot be excluded without a barium enema.
   F. **Treatment** consists of radiologic reduction, which is effective in 80-90%. Radiographic reduction is contraindicated if there is peritoneal irritation or toxicity.

V. **Midgut volvulus**
   A. Midgut volvulus results from the improper rotation and fixation of the duodenum

and colon (malrotation). Obstruction of the superior mesenteric artery may cause ischemic necrosis of the gut, which may be fatal.

- B. Infants in the first month constitute the majority of the cases. Symptoms usually begin about 5 days before diagnosis. The first sign of volvulus is bilious vomiting, followed by abdominal distention and GI bleeding. Peritonitis, hypovolemia, and shock may follow.
- C. **Abdominal x-ray** reveals a classic double bubble caused by duodenal obstruction. Pneumatosis intestinalis or distal bowel obstruction may also be apparent.
- D. Infants with rapid deterioration and obstructed loops of bowel require immediate surgery.
- E. If the infant is not critically ill, an UGI series with water-soluble, non-ionic, isoosmolar contrast will confirm midgut volvulus. If malrotation or volvulus (beak, spiral or corkscrew sign) is found, an immediate laparotomy is necessary.

VI. Gallbladder disease
- A. **Cholecystitis** in children occurs most commonly in the adolescent female, but it may affect infants who are only a few weeks of age. Cholecystitis is suggested by RUQ pain, back pain, or epigastric pain, radiating to the right subscapular area, bilious vomiting, fever, RUQ tenderness, and a RUQ mass. Jaundice is present in 25-55%, usually in association with hemolytic disease.
- B. **Ultrasonography** delineates gallstones and is the study of choice to screen for gallbladder disease.
- C. **Radioisotopic** scanning evaluates biliary and gallbladder function.

VII. Ectopic pregnancy
- A. Ectopic pregnancy must be considered in any postmenarchal, sexually active adolescent with abdominal pain. It is uncommon and usually seen in late adolescence. Ectopic pregnancy occurs in 0.5-3% of all pregnancies.
- B. Signs of ectopic pregnancy include abdominal pain in any location, vaginal bleeding, and/or amenorrhea. Nausea and vomiting, other symptoms of pregnancy, and lightheadedness may also be present.
- C. Abdominal, adnexal, and/or cervical tenderness are often found on pelvic examination, but occasionally abdominal tenderness is absent. The cervix may be soft (Godell's sign) and bluish in color (Chadwick's sign). The examination may reveal adnexal fullness and uterine enlargement.
- D. Evaluation includes a pregnancy test and ultrasound. Treatment consists of removal of the ectopic pregnancy by laparoscopy or exploratory laparotomy.

VIII. Gonadal pain in males
- A. In males with lower abdominal pain, the scrotum and its contents must be examined. Testicular torsion is a surgical emergency and must be treated within 6 hours of the onset of the pain to save the testicle.
- B. Testicular torsion may present as lower abdominal pain, which may be associated with recent trauma or cold. The gonad is tender and elevated in the scrotum, with a transverse orientation. Although testicular torsion may occur at any age, it usually occurs in adolescent males at puberty or shortly afterwards. It may occur in neonates. If the scrotum is empty, then torsion of a testicle located in the groin or in the abdomen should be ruled out.

IX. Gonadal pain in females
- A. The leading causes of gonadal pain in females are ovarian cysts and torsion of uterine adnexal structures. Ovarian tumors are often associated with precocious puberty or virilization.
- B. **Ovarian cysts** are responsible for 25% of childhood ovarian tumors, most commonly in adolescents. Bleeding into the cyst or cystic rupture causes pain,

which usually subsides within 12-24 hours. Ultrasound may show pelvic fluid and the cyst.

C. **Torsion of uterine adnexal structures**
  1. Torsion is associated with unilateral, sudden, severe pain with nausea and vomiting. The patient may also have subacute or chronic symptoms, with intermittent pain for days. The pain is usually diffuse and periumbilical in younger patients, but in older children and adolescents, the pain may radiate initially to the anterior thigh or ipsilateral groin.
  2. Fever and leucocytosis are usually present. Physical exam may reveal muscle rigidity and fixation of the mass on pelvic examination.
  3. Ultrasound will identify the mass accurately.
  4. Surgical exploration may sometimes salvage the ovary. Malignant neoplasms may cause torsion in 35% of cases.

X. **Meckel diverticulum**
  A. Meckel diverticulum are present in 2% of the population. It presents as a tender left lower quadrant mass, associated with blood in the stool.
  B. Vague abdominal pain with hemoccult positive stools suggests a Meckel Diverticulum. Bleeding is seen in 35-40% of childhood cases. A technetium nuclear scan may confirm the diagnosis.

References, see page 182.

Recurrent Abdominal Pain

Recurrent abdominal pain (RAP) is defined as paroxysmal abdominal pain in children between the ages of 4 and 16 years that persists for more than 3 months and affects normal activity. RAP is not a diagnosis. RAP is usually caused by a functional bowel disorder, and no specific cause can be determined. Functional abdominal pain is a diagnosis of exclusion.

I. **Clinical presentation**
  A. Children who have RAP exhibit one of three presentations: 1) isolated paroxysmal abdominal pain, 2) abdominal pain associated with symptoms of dyspepsia, and 3) abdominal pain associated with an altered bowel pattern. The pathogenesis of the pain may involve disordered gastrointestinal motility or visceral hypersensitivity. Most children "outgrow" the pain symptoms.
  B. Pain typically is periumbilical in location and variable in severity. Pain episodes tend to cluster, alternating with pain-free periods. Gastrointestinal symptoms are usually denied. Pain episodes begin gradually and last less than 1 hour. The child usually is unable to describe the pain.

II. **Differential diagnosis**
  A. **Fecal impaction** should be suspected if a left lower quadrant mass or suprapubic fullness is palpated, if the rectal examination reveals evidence of firm stool in the rectal vault, or if perianal soiling is present.
  B. **Parasitic infections** (Giardia lamblia, Blastocystis hominis, Dientamoeba fragilis) may present with chronic pain in the absence of altered bowel pattern.
  C. **Partial small bowel obstruction** may cause recurrent abdominal pain, associated with anorexia, nausea, and weight loss.
  D. **Crohn disease** should be suspected when tenderness is localized to the right lower quadrant, a fullness or mass effect is appreciated on abdominal examination, and fever, rash, or joint pains are present.

E. **Ureteropelvic junction obstruction** rarely may present with recurrent episodes of periumbilical or midepigastric crampy pain associated with episodic vomiting. Urinalysis may reveal microscopic hematuria.

F. **Appendiceal colic** should be suspected in recurrent acute, well-localized abdominal pain and tenderness, most commonly in the right lower quadrant.

G. **Dysmenorrhea** consists of cramping, dull, midline, or generalized lower abdominal pain at the onset of the menstrual period.

H. **Muscle pain** usually is well localized and sharp and may be triggered by exercise or a change in body position. It usually is located near the insertion of the rectus muscle or oblique muscles into the costal margins or iliac crest.

I. **Abdominal migraine and acute intermittent porphyria** (AIP) are characterized by paroxysmal abdominal pain and CNS symptoms, including headache, dizziness, weakness, syncope, confusion, memory loss, hallucinations, seizures, and transient blindness. Abdominal migraine is associated with cyclic vomiting. AIP often is precipitated by low intake of carbohydrate or by barbiturates or sulfonamides. A positive family history of these disorders is common.

J. **Psychogenic abdominal pain** that is triggered by environmental stress or critical life setbacks suggests a conversion reaction. Factors suggesting a conversion reaction include age at onset greater than 12 years, hysterical personality (dramatic, exhibitionist, labile, excitable), and a parent who is depressed.

Differential Diagnosis of Recurrent Abdominal Pain

- Functional abdominal pain
- Fecal impaction
- Parasitic infection
- Partial small bowel obstruction
  - Crohn disease
  - Malrotation with or without volvulus
  - Intussusception
  - Postsurgical adhesions
  - Small bowel lymphoma
  - Infection (tuberculosis, Yersinia)
  - Eosinophilic gastroenteritis
  - Angioneurotic edema
- Ureteropelvic junction obstruction
- Appendiceal colic
- Dysmenorrhea
  - Endometriosis
  - Ectopic pregnancy
  - Adhesions from pelvic inflammatory disease
- Cystic teratoma of ovary
- Musculoskeletal disorders
  - Muscle pain
  - Linea alba hernia
  - Discitis
- Vascular disorders
  - Mesenteric thrombosis
  - Polyarteritis nodosa
- Abdominal migraine
- Acute intermittent porphyria
- Psychiatric disorders

III. Diagnosis

A. Results of the physical examination, including rectal examination, are usually normal. The behavior, affect, and activity of the child are usually inconsistent with the degree of expressed pain. Poorly localized pressure tenderness frequently is elicited during abdominal palpation.

B. Laboratory evaluation should screen for occult inflammatory conditions, urinary tract infection, and parasitic infection. Testing may include a CBC, sedimentation rate, urinalysis, urine culture, and stool ovum and parasites.

Diagnostic Criteria for Functional Abdominal Pain

- Documentation of chronicity
- Compatible age range, age of onset
- Characteristic features of abdominal pain
- Evidence of physical or psychological stressful stimuli
- Environmental reinforcement of pain behavior
- Normal physical examination (including rectal examination and stool guaiac)
- Normal laboratory evaluation (CBC, sedimentation rate, urinalysis, urine culture, stool ovum and parasites)

"Red Flags" that Suggest an Organic Cause of Functional Abdominal Pain

- Pain awakening the child at night
- Localized pain away from the umbilicus
- Involuntary weight loss or growth deceleration
- Extraintestinal symptoms (fever, rash, joint pain, recurrent aphthous ulcers, dysuria)
- Consistent sleepiness following attacks of pain
- Blood in stools (guaiac-positive)
- Anemia
- Elevated ESR
- Positive family history of peptic ulcer disease, inflammatory bowel disease

---

IV. Treatment of recurrent abdominal pain

A. **Environmental modification** is the primary treatment for functional abdominal pain. Stresses that may provoke pain should be eliminated. Reinforcement of the pain behavior should cease. Lifestyle must be normalized and regular school attendance assured. The family should direct less attention toward the symptoms.

B. **A high-fiber diet or bulk-producing agents** may be useful if there is associated constipation.

C. **Avoiding excessive intake of milk products (lactose)**, carbonated beverages (fructose), dietary starches (corn, potatoes, wheat, oats), or sorbitol-containing products (vehicle for oral medication, sugar substitute in gum and candy, toothpaste, and gelatin capsules) may provide some relief. Confirmation of lactose intolerance by a lactose breath hydrogen test should be considered before recommending prolonged lactase enzyme replacement therapy or lactose-free milk products.

D. **Antispasmodics** may bring clinical improvement when given for a finite period of time.

E. **Consultation with a child psychiatrist or psychologist** may be indicated when there is concern about: 1) conversion reaction; 2) anxiety, depression, low self-esteem; 3) modeling or imitating family pain; 4) maladaptive family coping mechanisms; or 5) initial attempts at environmental modification not resulting in relief.

References, see page 182.

Chronic Nonspecific Diarrhea

Diarrhea is considered chronic when it persists for longer than 3 weeks. Chronic nonspecific diarrhea (CNSD) presents in toddlers between 18 months and 3 years of age, with frequent, large, watery stools in the absence of physical or laboratory signs of malabsorption or infection and without effect on growth or development. Children have 3 to 6, large, watery bowel movements daily. The diarrhea spontaneously resolves in 90% of children by 40 months of age.

I. **Pathogenesis**
    A. **Factors causing CNSD**
        1. Excess fluid intake
        2. Carbohydrate malabsorption from excessive juice ingestion
        3. Disordered intestinal motility
        4. Excessive fecal bile acids
        5. Low fat intake
    B. CNSD occurs when fluid intake exceeds the absorptive capacity of the intestinal tract. Malabsorption of carbohydrates (sucrose, fructose, sorbitol) in fruit juices contributes to CNSD.
    C. CNSD presents between 18 months and 3 years, with 3-6 large, loose, watery stools per day for more than 3 weeks.
    D. Stooling is most frequent in the morning and does not occur during sleep. There is an absence of nausea, vomiting, abdominal pain, flatulence, blood, fever, anorexia, weight loss, or poor growth.
II. **Clinical evaluation of chronic nonspecific diarrhea**
    A. The current number and type of stools should be determined. A diet history should determine the total calories, fat, milk and juice consumed daily, and it should assess prior trials of food elimination.
    B. The timing of introduction of foods into the diet relative to the onset of diarrhea, and a 3-day diet history should be assessed. Usage of antibiotics, vitamins, iron, and medications should be sought.
    C. A family history of irritable bowel syndrome, celiac disease, inflammatory bowel disease, infectious diarrhea, or food allergies should be sought.
    D. **Physical examination**
        1. Growth chart plotting of weight, height, and head circumference are essential. Children who have CNSD should continue to grow normally; deviation from the growth chart or a downward trend suggests inadequate caloric intake or a disease other than CNSD.
        2. Signs of malnutrition or malabsorption include lack of subcutaneous fat, eczematoid rash (from essential fatty acid deficiency), glossitis, easy bruising, or hyporeflexia.
    E. **Laboratory tests**
        1. A fresh stool specimen is tested for neutral fat with an oil stain, pH and reducing substances, occult blood, and Giardia antigen. Neutral fat suggest pancreatic insufficiency.

2. Fecal pH and reducing substances will reveal carbohydrate malabsorption if the pH is less than 5.5 or if reducing substances are greater than 1+.
3. Occult fecal blood is inconsistent with CNSD unless there is a perianal rash.
4. Giardia and Cryptosporidium are common and should be excluded with 3 stool samples for ova and parasites.

Stool Evaluation		
Test	Result	Disease
pH	<5.5	Carbohydrate malabsorption
Reducing substances	>1+	
Neutral fat	>40 globules/high power field	Pancreatic insufficiency
Occult blood	Positive	Enteritis or colitis
Giardia antigen	Positive	Giardiasis
Ova and parasites	Positive	Giardiasis, crypto-sporidiosis

III. Differential diagnosis

A. The differential diagnosis of chronic diarrhea in the 6-to 36-month-old child includes disaccharidase deficiency, protein intolerance, enteric infection, and malabsorption.

B. **Lactase deficiency**
1. **Lactase deficiency** may cause diarrhea associated with milk ingestion. In toddlers it is usually is caused by viral gastroenteritis.
2. **Lactose intolerance** caused by acute viral gastroenteritis usually resolves within 10-14 days.
3. **Congenital lactase deficiency** is extremely rare and symptoms are present from birth if an infant is fed human milk or a lactose-containing formula.
4. **Genetically acquired lactase deficiency** is common, but it usually is not symptomatic before 5 years of age.

C. **Congenital sucrase-isomaltase deficiency** is rare, producing symptoms when sucrose-containing formula or foods are introduced.

D. **Disaccharidase deficiency** can be confirmed by eliminating the specific carbohydrate or by breath hydrogen analysis after ingestion of lactose or sucrose.

E. **Milk-induced colitis** occurs in infants younger than 1 year of age who typically appear healthy but lose blood in their stool after ingesting milk protein. Infants who have milk-induced enterocolitis are younger, less than 3 months of age. These infants may be severely ill with bloody diarrhea, hypoproteinemia, and growth failure. Children who have protein allergies tend to come from families that have allergic histories, and affected children may have other atopic disorders (eczema, allergic rhinitis, asthma).

F. **Giardia or Cryptosporidium enteric infections** are commonly transmitted by asymptomatic carriers at child care centers. Foul-smelling diarrhea usually is associated with abdominal distension and flatus. Diagnosis is confirmed Giardia antigen in stool or three stools for ova and parasites.

G. **Malabsorption** presents with chronic diarrhea, weight loss, poor appetite, weakness and decreased activity, bloating and flatulence, abdominal pain, and chronic vomiting. The most common causes are cystic fibrosis and celiac disease. Chronic diarrhea and failure to thrive warrants a sweat test. Screening for celiac disease consists of a D-xylose absorption test and a serum celiac disease panel (antigliadin, antiendomysial, and antireticulin antibodies). Celiac disease must be confirmed by intestinal biopsy.

IV. Management of CNSD

A. Fluid intake should be gradually reduced to less than 100 mL/kg/day. Water is substituted for juice to reduce the child's interest in drinking. Switching from the bottle to the cup also decreases fluid intake.

B. Fat intake is increased to 4 g/kg/day by adding whole milk to the diet. If lactose intolerance is present, low-lactose milk can be used or lactase drops can be added to milk.

1. Butter, margarine, or vegetable oil are liberally added to foods for children less than 2 years of age.

C. Dietary fiber can be increased by consumption of fresh fruits and vegetables or by the addition of bran.

D. Removing dairy products to avoid lactose malabsorption may leave the child's diet with insufficient calories. Gluten-free diets and diets that restrict other proteins, such as cow milk protein, also should not be used without evidence of celiac disease, protein intolerance, or allergy.

References, see page 182.

Constipation

Constipation is common in infants and children. The problem usually resolves after modification of the child's fluid and dietary regimen.

I. Pathophysiology

A. Persistent difficulty with the passage of stool may lead to impaction, stool withholding, and fecal soiling.

Conditions Associated With Constipation	
Condition	**Common Causes**
Lack of Fecal Bulk	High-carbohydrate or high-protein diet Undernutrition
Abnormally Hard Stools	Excessive cow milk intake
Abnormally Dry Stools	Dehydration Infantile renal acidosis Diabetes insipidus Idiopathic hypercalcemia

Condition	Common Causes
Nervous System Lesion	Spinal cord lesions
Mechanical Obstruction	Anorectal stenotic lesions Intrinsic and extrinsic masses Strictures Aganglionosis (Hirschsprung disease)
Diseases That Complicate Defecation	Amyotonia congenita Cerebral palsy Hypertonia Hypothyroidism

II. **Neonates and infants younger than 1 year of age**
   A. **Evaluation**
      1. Inadequate fluid intake, undernutrition, and excessive cow milk intake should be excluded during the history.
      2. Anal inspection at the time of birth reveals anorectal anomalies in one in every 2,500 live births. Anal stenosis accounts for 20% of these abnormalities. The anus appears very small with a central black dot of meconium, and the infant must make an intense effort to pass a ribbon-like stool. The abdomen may be distended and stool can often be palpated on abdominal examination.
      3. **Hirschsprung disease**
         a. Hirschsprung disease accounts for 20-25% of cases of neonatal obstruction, and it is more common in males. Symptoms develop during the first month of life in 80%. The majority of infants are unable to pass stool normally during the first week.
         b. Infants with Hirschsprung disease usually fail to pass meconium during the first 48 hours of life. The abdomen is usually distended and tympanitic. Abdominal peristaltic activity may be visible, and fecal masses may be palpable. The anal canal and rectum are empty of feces, and the rectum is often narrow.
         c. Plain abdominal radiographs reveal gas and stool in the colon above the rectum. A rectosigmoid index (the diameter of the rectum divided by the diameter of the sigmoid) of less than one is consistent with Hirschsprung disease.
         d. When findings from the history, physical, and plain abdominal radiographs suggest Hirschsprung disease, contrast examination of the unprepared colon should be obtained. The diagnosis is confirmed by endoscopic biopsy.
   B. **Management of simple constipation in infants**
      1. Dietary corrective measures are the initial therapy for infants with simple constipation. Increasing fluid intake and the percentage of calories from carbohydrates often corrects the problem. Barley malt extract is often helpful.
      2. Infants that do not respond to dietary measures are treated with a mineral oil preparation. Routine suppository administration, enemas, and stimulant laxatives should be avoided.

III. Older infants and children
A. Evaluation
1. Fluid and dietary fiber intake should be assessed. Older children with chronic constipation and stool withholding activity usually also have fecal incontinence because unformed stool passes around the impaction and leaks out of the anus.
2. A complete physical examination should exclude systemic illnesses that might be complicated by constipation. Moveable fecal masses are often appreciated in the left colon and sigmoid.
3. The lower back should be examined for a deep pilonidal dimple with hair tuft and/or sacral agenesis, suggestive of myelodysplasia. Anal inspection may reveal primary anal disease. Normal anal tone found on rectal examination indicates normal anal innervation. The rectal vault may be filled with inspissated stool.
4. Anteroposterior and lateral x-rays of the abdomen usually reveal a large rectal/rectosigmoid impaction with variable amounts of stool throughout the remainder of the colon.

B. Management of chronic constipation
1. Distal impaction should be removed with hypertonic phosphate enemas (Fleet enema). Usually three enemas are administered during a 36- to 48-hour period.
2. **Mineral oil** should be prescribed. The initial dose of mineral oil is 30-75 mL (1-2.5 oz) twice daily. Mineral oil is tasteless, and it can be taken with fruit juice, Kool-Aid, or a soft drink. After one month, the oil is tapered by 15 mL (0.5 oz) per dose.
3. The child should sit on the toilet, with proper foot support, for five minutes after the evening meal to take advantage of the gastrocolic reflex in establishing a regular bowel pattern. A bulk-type stool softener (eg, Metamucil) should be initiated when the mineral oil dosage has been tapered to 15 mL twice daily.

References, see page 182.

Gastroenteritis

Acute gastroenteritis consists of as diarrheal disease of rapid onset, often with nausea, vomiting, fever, or abdominal pain. It occurs an average of 1.3-2.3 times per year between the ages of 0 and 5 years. Most episodes of acute gastroenteritis will resolve within 3 to 7 days.

I. Pathophysiology.
Gastroenteritis in children is caused by viral, bacterial, and parasitic organisms, although the vast majority of cases are viral or bacterial in origin. Oral ingestion is the primary route of infection, although rotavirus is transmitted by respiratory or mucous membrane contact as well.

II. Viral gastroenteritis
A. All of the viruses produce watery diarrhea often accompanied by vomiting and fever, but usually not associated with blood or leukocytes in the stool or with prominent cramping.
B. **Rotavirus** is the predominant viral cause of dehydrating diarrhea. Rotaviral infections tend to produce severe diarrhea, causing up to 70% of episodes in children under 2 years of age who require hospitalization. Rotavirus infection

tends to occur in the fall in the southwest of the US, then sweeping progressively eastward, reaching the northeast by late winter and spring.

C. **Norwalk viruses** are the major cause of large epidemics of acute nonbacterial gastroenteritis, occurring in schools, camps, nursing homes, cruise ships, and restaurants.

D. **Enteric adenovirus** is the third most common organism isolated in infantile diarrhea.

III. **Bacterial gastroenteritis**

A. The bacterial diarrheas are caused by elaboration of toxin (enterotoxigenic pathogens) or by invasion and inflammation of the mucosa (invasive pathogens).

B. **Secretory diarrheas** are modulated through an enterotoxin, and the patient does not have systemic symptoms (fever, myalgias) or signs of local irritation of the bowel (tenesmus), or evidence of gut inflammation in the stool (white or red blood cells). The diarrhea is watery, often is large in volume, and often associated with nausea and vomiting.

C. **Invasive diarrhea** is caused by bacterial enteropathogens, and is accompanied by systemic signs, such as fever, myalgias, arthralgias, irritability, and loss of appetite. Cramps and abdominal pain are prominent. The diarrhea consists of frequent passing of small amounts of "mucousy" stool. Stool examination reveals leukocytes, red blood cells, and often gross blood.

Acute Diarrhea Patterns and Associated Pathogens	
Secretory/enterotoxigenic	**Inflammatory**
Characterized by watery diarrhea and absence of fecal leukocytes	Characterized by dysentery (ie, fever and bloody stools), fecal leukocytes, and erythrocytes
Food poisoning (toxigenic)	
Staphylococcus aureus *Bacillus cereus* *Clostridium perfringens*	*Shigella* Invasive *E coli* *Salmonella* *Campylobacter*
Enterotoxigenic	
Escherichia coli *Vibrio cholera* *Giardia lamblia* *Cryptosporidium* Rotavirus Norwalk-like virus	*C difficile* *Entameba histolytica*

IV. **General approach to the patient with gastroenteritis**

A. **Determining and managing the fluid losses, dehydration and electrolyte abnormalities** is more important than ascertaining the specific microbiologic cause.

B. **History** should assess recent antibiotic use, underlying diseases, other illnesses in the family, travel, untreated water, raw shellfish, attendance at a child care center, and foods eaten recently.

Clinical Evaluation and Treatment of Acute Diarrhea

Step One--Assess child for degree of dehydration

No dehydration	Continue oral hydration and feeding
Mild/severe dehydration-------->	Initiate rehydration by oral route (intravenous for severely dehydrated patients)

Step Two--Assess Clinical History for Etiologic Clues

Etiologic Clue	Etiology Suggested
Fever, crampy abdominal pain, tenesmus	Inflammatory colitis or ileitis
History of bloody stool	Shigella, enteroinvasive E coli, amebiasis, other bacterial causes
Fever and abdominal pain	Yersinia enterocolitis
Current or previous antibiotic use	Antibiotic-associated enteritis or pseudomembranous colitis
Multiple cases and common food source	Incubation <6 hours: Staphylococcus aureus, Bacillus cereus Incubation >6 hours: Clostridium perfringens
Ingestion of inadequately cooked seafood	Vibrio parahaemolyticus
Recent measles, severe malnutrition, AIDS, other causes of immunosuppression	Bacterial (Salmonella), viral (rotavirus), or parasitic (isosporiasis, Cryptosporidium)

Step Three--Examine Stool:

	Indicated for:	Finding:	Etiology Suggested:
Visual examination	All patients	Gross blood	Dysentery, colitis, invasive organism
Microscopic examination for white/red blood cells	Patients who have had diarrhea >3 days, fever, blood in stool, weight loss	Red cells and leukocytes Red cells without leukocytes	Shigella, enterohemorrhagic EC, enteroinvasive EC, Campylobacter, Clostridium, E histolytica
Parasitic examination (wet mount, acid-fast staining, or concentration)	Diarrhea >10 days	Positive	Giardia, Amoeba, Cryptosporidium, Isospora, Strongyloides
Clostridium difficile toxin	Patients taking antibiotics	Positive	C difficile colitis

Assessment of Diarrheal Dehydration					
Clinical Finding	Mild (10-40 mL/kg)	Moderate (50-90 mL/kg)			Severe (100-130 mL/kg)
Affect/sensorium	Normal	Irritability		Lethargy	Stupor
Eyes	Normal		Sunken		Deeply sunken
Mucous membrane	Normal		Dry		Very dry
Tears when crying	Yes		No		No
Thirst	Normal	50	0	+++	++++ or unresponsive
Skin turgor (capillary refill)	Normal		Reduced (<1 sec)		Very reduced (2-3 sec)
Fontanelle	Normal		Depressed		Severely depressed
Pulse	Full	Full		Weak	Feeble or absent
Pulse rate	Normal		Elevated		Very rapid
Blood pressure	Normal		Normal		Low or absent

C. **Fluid therapy**
  1. **Mild-to-moderate dehydration**
     a. **Mildly or moderately dehydrated children** should receive oral rehydration therapy (ORT) at 50 mL/kg (mild dehydration) or 100 mL/kg (moderate dehydration) over a 4-hour period. Replacement of stool losses (at 10 mL/kg for each stool) and of emesis (estimated volume) will require adding appropriate amounts of solution to the total. If all but sips of fluid are vomited, oral hydration can be achieved by administering a teaspoonful of solution every 2 to 5 minutes.
     b. Use of cola, fruit juice and sports beverages are not recommended; their electrolyte content is inappropriate, and they contain too much carbohydrate.
  2. **Prevention of dehydration.** Children who have diarrhea, but not dehydrated, may be given glucose-electrolyte solution in addition to their regular diets to replace stool losses. The well-hydrated child should continue to consume an age-appropriate diet and drink more than the usual amounts of the normal fluids in his diet.
  3. **Severely dehydrated children** who are in a state of shock must receive immediate and aggressive intravenous (IV) therapy. When the patient is stable, hydration may be continued orally.
  4. **Intravenous rehydration**
     a. When intravenous rehydration is required, it should begin with an isotonic solution (normal saline, lactated Ringer). Severe dehydration clinically is associated with a loss of 10-12% of body weight in fluids and

electrolytes (100 to 120 mL/kg); therefore, this amount plus additional losses should be infused.

    b. Infusion rates of up to 100 mL/min are appropriate in older children. Infusion rates of 40 mL/kg are given over the first 30 minutes, with the remainder of the deficit (70 mL/kg) over the next 2.5 hours, until the calculated fluid loss has been replenished.

    c. For infants, correction should be slower, with infusion rates no more than 30 mL/kg over the first hour and the remaining 70 mL/kg over 5 hours.

    d. Subsequent maintenance fluids should be given orally. Oral fluids should be initiated as soon as the patient can drink. They should be given simultaneously with intravenous fluids until the total fluids administered have replenished the calculated deficit.

D. Antibiotic therapy

    1. The effectiveness of antimicrobial therapy is well established in shigellosis. Shigella is the cause of bacterial dysentery and is the second most commonly identified bacterial pathogen in diarrhea between the ages of 6 months and 10 years.

    2. It causes watery diarrhea with mucus and gross blood. Treatment usually consists of ceftriaxone or cefixime.

E. Refeeding

    1. Children who have diarrhea and are not dehydrated should continue to be fed age-appropriate diets. Fatty foods and foods high in simple sugars, such as sweetened tea, juices, and soft drinks should be avoided. Well-tolerated foods include complex carbohydrates (rice, wheat, potatoes, bread, cereals), lean meats, yogurt, fruits, and vegetables. The BRAT diet (bananas, rice, applesauce, toast) does not supply optimal nutrition.

    2. Introducing the child's regular form of milk early in the course of therapy is recommended.

F. Antidiarrheal compounds (eg, loperamide, diphenoxylate, bismuth compounds, Kaopectate) should not be used to treat acute diarrhea.

V. Laboratory examinations

A. Most noninflammatory diarrheal illnesses respond in 3 to 5 days to simple rehydration therapy and dietary management alone, obviating the need for initial laboratory evaluations. The presence of blood in the stool, fever, or persistence of the diarrhea for more than 3 days may trigger a laboratory pursuit of an etiologic agent.

B. Microscopic stool examination. If erythrocytes and white blood cells are present, particularly in the setting of fever, a bacterial pathogen (Campylobacter, Yersinia, Salmonella, Shigella) should be suspected. Many red blood cells in the absence of white blood cells suggests the presence of Entamoeba.

C. Stool culture should be reserved for individuals whose diarrhea has not responded to fluid and feeding and for those who have signs of inflammatory disease (fever, myalgias) and the presence of leukocytes or red blood cells in the stool.

References, see page 182.

Gastroesophageal Reflux

I. **Clinical evaluation of gastroesophageal reflux disease**
   A. **Infants.** Regurgitation is the classic symptom of gastroesophageal reflux (GERD) in infancy. However, infantile regurgitation is not always GERD and GERD may occur without any regurgitation.

Symptoms of Reflux
Symptoms due to regurgitation
Emesis with weight loss
Symptoms due to esophagitis Chest pain, irritability, feeding problems Anemia, hematemesis Esophageal obstruction due to stricture
Respiratory symptoms Pneumonia (especially recurrent or chronic) Wheezing, bronchospasm (especially intractable asthma) Apnea, cyanotic episodes (especially obstructive apnea) Miscellaneous: stridor, cough, hiccups, hoarseness Complex respiratory disease-reflux interactions --Esophageal atresia and tracheoesophageal fistula --Cystic fibrosis --Bronchopulmonary dysplasia
Neurobehavioral symptoms Infant "spells" (including seizure-like events) Sandifer syndrome

   B. **Children.** During the second or third year of life, pain, particularly substernal or epigastric, becomes more common than regurgitation as a presenting symptom for GERD. Heartburn suggests the presence of esophagitis.

II. **Management of mild symptoms of reflux**
   A. **Infants.** Mild reflux affects most infants in the form of regurgitation; 40% of healthy infants regurgitate more than once a day. This nonpathogenic regurgitation does not produce weight deficit, is not accompanied by abnormal irritability or other behaviors suggesting esophagitis, and is not associated with respiratory disease or apnea. It generally begins after the first few weeks of life, peaks at about 4 months of age, and resolves by 8 to 12 months of age as the diet becomes more solid.
   B. **Exposure of tobacco smoke** should be avoided because it induces lower esophageal sphincter relaxation
   C. **Seated and supine positions** provoke reflux. The seated position should be avoided, and the supine position should not be used for awake, observed times.

    D. Thickening of formula with 1 Tbsp of dry rice cereal per 1 oz of formula and using a cross-cut nipple that is slit with a razor blade reduces regurgitation. The bottle should be filled up so that air is not ingested.

    E. If there is a family history of allergy, a 2-week trial of an elemental formula will clarify whether cow milk allergy is playing any role. (The use of a soy formula as a diagnostic trial is not helpful because of the frequency of concurrent sensitivity to both cow milk and soy.) For breast-fed infants, the mother may try eliminating cow milk protein from her diet.

III. Diagnostic testing

    A. Infants. Barium radiography evaluates the anatomy; scintigraphy will detect delayed gastric emptying or aspiration. A pH probe assesses the temporal association of reflux episodes with symptoms.

Treatment of Reflux

Conservative, life-style changes
Position: Avoid supine and seated positions for awake infants
Thicken infant feedings: 1 Tbsp dry rice cereal per 1 oz formula
Avoid feeding before bedtime
Avoid large meals, obesity, tight clothing
Avoid foods and medications that lower esophageal sphincter tone or increase gastric acidity
Fatty foods, citrus, tomato, carbonated drinks, coffee, alcohol, acidic beverages, tobacco smoke
Anticholinergics, adrenergics, xanthines (theophylline, caffeine), calcium channel blockers, prostaglandins

Pharmacologic therapy (usual course is 8 weeks)
Prokinetic:
    Cisapride (Propulsid) 0.2 mg/kg per dose QID: before meal, before bed; maximum 10 mg QID
Antacid:
    Cimetidine (Tagamet) 10 mg/kg per dose QID: before meal, before bed; maximum 300 mg QID
    Antacids (0.5 to 1 mL/kg per dose, 3 to 8 times per day: 1 to 2 h after meal, before bed)
    Use magnesium-containing antacids for constipated children and the "gel" antacids for those whose stools are loose.

Surgical
    Fundoplication
    Gastrojejunostomy feedings (also usually require pharmacotherapy)

    B. For the infant who has GERD, it is useful to begin with conservative measures, add cisapride (Propulsid) when the diagnosis of GERD is diagnosed, and add a histamine-2 (H2) blocker when esophagitis is established. Cimetidine (Tagamet) is the optimal H2 blocker for pediatric GERD because it is inexpensive, has an identical dosing schedule to cisapride, and has better-established pediatric dosing requirements. Pharmacotherapy generally is discontinued by 12 months of age.

References, see page 182.

Inflammatory Bowel Disease

I. **Initial evaluation of chronic diarrhea**
   A. **The initial diagnostic evaluation** of chronic diarrhea includes stool cultures for enteric pathogens, tests for ova and parasites, Clostridium difficile toxin, and fecal leukocytes. Specific cultures for Yersinia enterocolitica, isolation of toxigenic strains of Escherichia coli, and serologic titers for Entamoeba histolytica may also be necessary.
   B. **Laboratory studies** to assess disease activity and nutritional state include levels of C-reactive protein, which correlates with severity of disease, and levels of serum proteins (eg, albumin, transferrin, prealbumin, retinol-binding protein), which assess nutritional status. The degree of anemia indicates the severity of mucosal injury and duration of illness.
   C. **Colonoscopy or flexible sigmoidoscopy** with biopsy is valuable in character-izing mucosal injury.
   D. **Abdominal plain films** with the patient in upright and supine positions should be obtained in patients with severe disease to detect perforation, toxic megacolon, or thumbprinting.

II. **Ulcerative colitis**
   A. Ulcerative colitis (UC) is the most common cause of chronic colitis. The pathogenesis remain unknown. Inflammation is localized primarily in the mucosa. The most common symptoms are abdominal pain, rectal bleeding, diarrhea, fever, and malaise.
   B. The incidence ranges from 4 to 15 cases per 100,000. Disease may present at any time but does so most often during adolescence and young adulthood, with a higher risk of the disease in young females than males. Among family members, the risk is tenfold higher. Ashkenazi Jews are afflicted more often than non-Jewish populations.
   C. Thirty percent of UC patients present with disease limited to the rectum, 40% have more extensive disease but not extending beyond the hepatic flexure, and 30% have total colonic involvement.
   D. **Diagnostic evaluation**
      1. Inflammation characteristically begins in the rectum. The mucosa is erythematous, friable, and edematous, with superficial erosions and ulcerations. Histologic features of ulcerative colitis include diffuse shallow ulceration of the mucosa, crypt abscesses, thickening of the muscularis mucosa, and pronounced inflammatory cell infiltration.
      2. **Extraintestinal manifestations**
         a. **Musculoskeletal.** Arthritis is the most common extraintestinal manifes-tation of ulcerative colitis. It is migratory, often involving the hip, ankle, wrist, or elbow. It is usually monoarticular and asymmetric, and its course parallels that of the colitis. Ankylosing spondylitis and sacroiliitis, or axial arthritis, typically present as low back pain with morning stiffness.
         b. **Ocular.** Episcleritis, uveitis, and iritis may occur.
         c. **Dermatologic.** Abnormalities may include erythema nodosum, pyoderma gangrenosum, lichen planus, and aphthous ulcers.

        d. Hepatobiliary. Manifestations may include hepatic steatosis, primary sclerosing cholangitis (4%), cholelithiasis, and pericholangitis.

        e. Miscellaneous. Other complications include nephrolithiasis and a hypercoagulable state.

III. Crohn disease

A. Crohn disease (CD) is a chronic inflammatory process, which may involve any portion of the gastrointestinal tract from the mouth to the anus. Inflammation is characterized by transmural extension and irregular involvement of the intestinal tract, with intervening normal tissue ("skip areas"). Most often, the distal ileum and proximal colon are involved; in about 25% of cases, only the colon is affected.

B. Crohn disease often has its onset during adolescence and young adulthood. It is more common in females. The overall risk is two to four times higher in first-degree relatives.

C. Fever, abdominal pain, diarrhea, weight loss, and fatigue are common. Rectal bleeding is not as prominent a feature in Crohn disease as it is in ulcerative colitis. About 20% of patients have evidence of perianal disease, such as perirectal fistulas, anal skin tags, anal ulcerations or fissures, or perirectal abscesses. Crohn disease causes extra-intestinal manifestations like those of ulcerative colitis.

D. Diagnostic evaluation

    1. Anemia, caused by chronic blood loss, and a mildly elevated white blood cell count are common.

    2. Endoscopic findings include focal ulcerations and inflammation is interrupted by skip areas. Other features of Crohn disease include rectal sparing, cobblestone appearance, strictures, and ileal involvement. Biopsies can confirm the presence of skip areas and granulomatous inflammation.

IV. Management of ulcerative colitis

A. Mild-to-moderate cases of ulcerative colitis

    1. The oral 5-ASA compound, mesalamine (Asacol) is used for active ulcerative colitis, and olsalazine sodium (Dipentum) is used for maintenance therapy. The target dosage for the tablet Asacol (in divided doses) is 2.4 g/day, the capsule (Pentasa) 4 g/day, and capsule olsalazine (Dipentum) 1 g/day.

    2. Limited left-sided colonic disease or rectosigmoid disease may respond to local therapy (enemas, suppositories) with corticosteroids and mesalamine.

    3. Rectal preparations of mesalamine (Rowasa enema and suppository) can deliver higher concentrations to the distal colon for proctitis. Rowasa (4 g) is the only enema preparation of 5-ASA.

B. Moderately severe cases of ulcerative colitis

    1. These patients may require rehydration or blood transfusion. Corticosteroids, a low-residue diet, and local therapy should be initiated.

    2. Prednisone usually is started at a dose of 1 to 2 mg/kg per day for 1 to 2 weeks. Once the patient has stabilized, the patient is weaned off the steroids to alternate-day therapy over 4 to 8 weeks; aminosalicylates usually are started before the steroid taper is begun. The rectal corticosteroid preparation, hydrocortisone retention enema (Cortenema), is effective for distal ulcerative colitis.

C. Fulminant ulcerative colitis requires immediate hospitalization. Fluid and electrolyte status must be stabilized and blood transfusions given as needed. Intravenous corticosteroids (methylprednisolone), broad-spectrum antibiotics (metronidazole, an aminoglycoside, and ampicillin), parenteral nutrition, and

bowel rest are initiated.
- **D.** If the patient deteriorates clinically or develops complications (hemorrhage, toxic megacolon), emergency surgery is performed. If the patient has not improved for 2 to 4 weeks after maximal medical therapy, a colectomy should be considered. Surgery is curative for UC.
- **E.** Cyclosporine therapy has been used in severe cases; in adults, doses of 4 mg/kg per day resulted in improvement in 80% of patients. If the patient is steroid-dependent, 6-mercaptopurine or azathioprine can be used.

Treatment of Inflammatory Bowel Disease

	Dose/day	Route	Side Effects
5-Aminosalicylic Acid			
Mesalamine (Asacol)	30-50 mg/kg	PO	Nephrotoxicity
Mesalamine (Rowasa)			
Enema	2-4 g QD	PR	Chills, diarrhea
Suppository	500 mg BID	PR	Local irritation
Mesalamine (Pentasa)	50-60 mg/kg	PO	Nephrotoxicity
Olsalazine (Dipentum)	20-30 mg/kg	PO	Watery diarrhea
Steroids			
Prednisone	1-2 mg/kg	PO	Osteoporosis, hypertension, poor growth, obesity, hirsutism, cataracts, adrenal suppression
Methylprednisolone	0.8-1.6 mg/kg	PO	Same as for prednisone
Hydrocortisone			
Enema	100 mg QD-BID	PR	Local irritation
Foam	80 mg QD-BID	PR	Same as enema
Immunosuppressants			
6-mercaptopurine	1-1.5 mg/kg	PO	Pancreatitis, bone marrow suppression
Azathioprine	1.5-2 mg/kg	PO	Same as for 6-mercaptopurine
Cyclosporine	2-4 mg/kg	IV	Nephrotoxicity
	4-6 mg/kg	PO	Hirsutism, hypertension
Antibiotics			
Metronidazole	10-20 mg/kg	PO/IV	Peripheral neuropathy, metallic taste

	Dose/day	Route	Side Effects
Miscellaneous			
Folic acid	1 mg	PO	

V. **Management of Crohn disease.** Treatment is similar to that of ulcerative colitis. Corticosteroids and 5-aminosalicylic acid agents are the mainstays of therapy. Patients with severe colitis, massive weight loss, and significant systemic symptoms may need to be hospitalized. Prednisone can induce a remission in 70% of patients who have small bowel disease.

   A. **Antibiotics** (metronidazole and ciprofloxacin) are useful in mild-to-moderate CD and perianal disease.

   B. **Immunosuppressive agents.** Mercaptopurine and azathioprine are reserved for patients with continuous disease activity despite corticosteroid therapy. Cyclosporine may be beneficial in refractory patients.

   C. **Surgery** for Crohn disease is not curative. Indications include obstruction or intractable symptoms. Disease almost always recurs after surgery.

References, see page 182.

Persistent Vomiting

Vomiting is defined as the forceful expulsion of gastric contents through the mouth. Vomiting can be caused by a benign, self-limited process or it may be indicative of a serious underlying disorder.

I. **Pathophysiology of vomiting**

   A. Vomiting is usually preceded by nausea, increased salivation, and retching. It is distinct from regurgitation, which is characterized by passive movement of gastric contents into the esophagus.

   B. Projectile vomiting results from intense gastric peristaltic waves, usually secondary to gastric outlet obstruction caused by hypertrophic pyloric stenosis or pylorospasm.

   C. Retching often precedes vomiting and is characterized by spasmodic contraction of the expiratory muscles with simultaneous abdominal contraction. Nausea is an imminent desire to vomit, usually induced by visceral stimuli.

II. Clinical evaluation of vomiting

Etiology of Vomiting by Age

	Newborn	Infant	Older Child
Obstruction	Malrotation of bowel Volvulus Intestinal atresia Intestinal stenosis Meconium ileus Meconium plug Hirschsprung disease Imperforate anus Incarcerated hernia	Pyloric stenosis Foreign bodies Malrotation (volvulus) Duplication of alimentary tract Intussusception Meckel diverticulum Hirschsprung disease Incarcerated hernia	Intussusception Foreign bodies Malrotation (volvulus) Meckel diverticulum Hirschsprung disease Incarcerated hernia Adhesions
Gastrointestinal disorders (infectious/inflammatory)	Necrotizing enterocolitis Gastroesophageal reflux Paralytic ileus Peritonitis Milk allergy	Gastroenteritis Gastroesophageal reflux Pancreatitis Appendicitis Celiac disease Paralytic ileus Peritonitis	Gastroenteritis Peptic ulcer disease
Infectious disorders (nongastrointestinal)	Sepsis Meningitis	Sepsis Meningitis Otitis media Pneumonia Pertussis Hepatitis Urinary tract infection	Meningitis Otitis media Pharyngitis Pneumonia Hepatitis Urinary tract infection
Neurologic disorders	Hydrocephalus Kernicterus Subdural hematoma Cerebral edema	Hydrocephalus Subdural hematoma Intracranial hemorrhage Mass lesion (abscess, tumor)	Subdural hematoma Intracranial hemorrhage Brain tumor Other mass-occupying lesion Migraine Motion sickness Hypertensive encephalopathy
Metabolic and endocrine disorders	Inborn errors of metabolism: Urea cycle defects, galactosemia, disorders of organic acid metabolism Congenital adrenal hyperplasia Neonatal tetany	Inborn errors of metabolism Fructose intolerance Adrenal insufficiency Metabolic acidosis	Adrenal insufficiency Diabetic ketoacidosis

	Newborn	Infant	Older Child
Renal disorders	Obstructive uropathy Renal insufficiency	Obstructive uropathy Renal insufficiency	Obstructive uropathy Renal insufficiency
Toxins		Digoxin Iron	Digoxin Iron Lead Food poisoning
Other			Pregnancy Anorexia nervosa Bulimia Psychogenic etiology

A. **Clinical evaluation of vomiting in the neonate**
   1. **Bilious vomiting**
      a. Bilious vomiting, at any age, suggests intestinal obstruction or systemic infection. Anatomic abnormalities of the gastrointestinal tract that may present in the first week of life with bilious vomiting and abdominal distention include malrotation, volvulus, duplications of the bowel, bowel atresia, meconium plug, meconium ileus, incarcerated hernia, and aganglionosis (Hirschsprung disease).
   2. **Necrotizing enterocolitis**
      a. NEC is the most common inflammatory condition of the intestinal tract in the neonate. Symptoms of NEC include abdominal distention, bilious vomiting, and blood in the stool.
      b. The infant who has NEC also may present with nonspecific signs of systemic infection, such as lethargy, apnea, temperature instability, and shock. NEC occurs mainly in preterm infants, although 10% of affected newborns present at term.
   3. **Metabolic disorders**
      a. **Inborn errors of metabolism** should be considered in any acute neonatal illness, including persistent vomiting. Factors that suggest a metabolic disorder include early or unexplained death of a sibling, multiple spontaneous maternal abortions, or history of consanguinity.
      b. Associated features may include lethargy, hypotonia, and convulsions.
   4. **Neurologic disorders**. Central nervous system abnormalities, such as intracranial hemorrhage, hydrocephalus and cerebral edema, should be suspected in the neonate who has neurologic deficits, a rapid increase in head circumference, or an unexplained fall in hematocrit.
B. **Clinical evaluation of vomiting in infancy**
   1. **Pyloric stenosis**
      a. Pyloric stenosis is a major consideration in infants. Hypertrophy of the pylorus causes gastric outlet obstruction at the pyloric canal. Five percent of infants whose parents had pyloric stenosis develop this disorder. Males are affected more often than females, and firstborns are more likely to be affected than subsequent siblings.
      b. Symptoms of pyloric stenosis usually begin at age 2 to 3 weeks, but may occur at birth or present as late as 5 months. An olive-size mass may be palpable in the right upper quadrant. A metabolic alkalosis frequently results from the vomiting.

2. Gastroesophageal reflux

a. Gastroesophageal reflux (GER) is defined as retrograde movement of gastric contents into the esophagus. GER occurs in 65% of infants and is caused by inappropriate relaxation of the lower esophageal sphincter.

b. GER is considered "pathologic" if symptoms persist beyond 18 to 24 months and/or if significant complications develop, such as failure to thrive, recurrent episodes of bronchospasm and pneumonia, apnea, or reflux esophagitis.

c. Reflux esophagitis should be suspected when regurgitation is accompanied by irritability during feeding, refusal to feed, failure to thrive or occult blood in the stool.

3. Gastrointestinal allergy

a. Cow milk allergy is rare in infancy and early childhood and generally resolves by 2 to 3 years of age. Vomiting, diarrhea, colic and gastrointestinal loss of blood may occur.

b. Other manifestations may include anaphylaxis, atopic dermatitis, urticaria, angioedema, and wheezing.

III. Clinical evaluation of vomiting in childhood

A. Peptic ulcer

1. Peptic ulcer disease in early childhood is often associated with vomiting. Peptic ulcer disease should be suspected if there is a family history of ulcer disease, or if there is hematemesis or unexplained iron deficiency anemia.

2. Abdominal pain typically wakes the patient from sleep. There may be epigastric tenderness and occult blood in the stool.

B. Pancreatitis

1. Pancreatitis is a relatively rare cause of vomiting, but should be considered in the child who has sustained abdominal trauma. Patients usually complain of epigastric pain, which may radiate to the mid-back.

2. Other factors predisposing to pancreatitis include viral illnesses (mumps), drugs (steroids, azathioprine), congenital anomalies of the biliary or pancreatic ducts, cholelithiasis, hypertriglyceridemia, and a family history of pancreatitis.

C. Central nervous system disorders.
Persistent vomiting without other gastrointestinal or systemic complaints suggests an intracranial tumor or other lesions that increase intracranial pressure. Subtle neurologic findings (eg, ataxia, head tilt) should be assessed and a detailed neurologic examination should be performed.

IV. Physical examination of the child with persistent vomiting

A. Volume depletion often results from vomiting, manifesting as sunken fontanelles, decreased skin turgor, dry mouth, absence of tears, and decreased urine output.

B. Peritoneal irritation should be suspected when the child to keeps his knees drawn up or bends over. Abdominal distension, visible peristalsis, and increased bowel sounds suggests intestinal obstruction.

C. Abnormal masses, enlarged organs, guarding, or tenderness should be sought. A hypertrophic pylorus may manifest as a palpable "olive" in the right upper quadrant.

D. Intussusception is often associated with a tender, sausage-shaped mass in the right upper quadrant and an empty right lower quadrant (Dance sign).

E. Digital rectal exam. Decreased anal sphincter tone and large amounts of hard fecal material in the ampulla suggests fecal impaction. Constipation, increased rectal sphincter tone, and an empty rectal ampulla suggests Hirschsprung disease. Blood suggests an inflammatory disease or peptic ulcer disease.

V. **Laboratory evaluation**
   A. **Serum electrolytes should be obtained** when dehydration is suspected.
   B. **Urinalysis** may detect a urinary tract infection or suggest the presence of a metabolic disorder.
   C. **Plasma amino acids and urine organic acids** should be measured if metabolic disease is suspected because of recurrent, unexplained episodes of metabolic acidosis.
   D. **Serum ammonia should be obtained in cases of cyclic vomiting** to exclude a urea cycle defect.
   E. **Liver chemistries and serum ammonia and glucose levels** should be obtained if liver disease is suspected.
   F. **Serum amylase** is frequently elevated in patients who have acute pancreatitis. Serum lipase levels may be more helpful because they remain elevated for a number of days following an acute episode.

VI. **Imaging studies**
   A. **Ultrasonography** of the abdomen is the initial imaging test for suspected pyloric stenosis; however, two-thirds of vomiting infants will have a negative sonogram and will subsequently require an upper gastrointestinal series.
   B. **Plain radiographs of the abdomen**
      1. **Supine and upright or left lateral decubitus radiographic views** are necessary for detecting congenital anatomic malformations or obstructive lesions.
      2. **Air-fluid levels** suggest obstruction, although this finding is nonspecific and may be seen with gastroenteritis.
      3. **Free air** in the abdominal cavity indicates a perforated viscus. Upright plain films may demonstrate free air under the diaphragm; a left decubitus view will show air outlining the liver.
   C. **Upper gastrointestinal series** with nonionic, iso-osmolar, water-soluble contrast is indicated when anatomic abnormalities and/or conditions that cause gastric outlet obstruction are suspected.
   D. **Barium enema** should be performed to detect lower intestinal obstruction, and it may also be therapeutic in intussusception.
   E. **Endoscopy.** If radiographic studies are negative for intestinal obstruction, upper endoscopy should be considered in patients suspected of having inflammatory conditions of the proximal gastrointestinal tract, such as peptic ulcer disease, or reflux esophagitis.

VII. **Treatment**
   A. **Initial therapy** should correct hypovolemia and electrolyte abnormalities. In acute diarrheal illnesses with vomiting, oral rehydration therapy is usually adequate for treatment of dehydration.
   B. **Bilious vomiting and suspected intestinal obstruction** is managing by giving nothing by mouth, and by placing a nasogastric tube connected to intermittent suction. Bilious vomiting requires surgical consultation.
   C. **Pharmacologic therapy**
      1. **Antiemetic agents** usually are not required because most instances of acute vomiting are caused by self-limited, infectious gastrointestinal illnesses. Antiemetic drugs may be indicated for postoperative emesis, motion sickness, cytotoxic drug-evoked emesis, and gastroesophageal reflux disease.
      2. **Diphenhydramine and dimenhydrinate** are useful in treating the symptoms of motion sickness or vestibulitis.
      3. **Prochlorperazine and chlorpromazine** have anticholinergic and

antihistaminic properties and are used to treat vomiting caused by drugs, radiation, and gastroenteritis.

References, see page 182.

Neurologic and Rheumatic Disorders

Febrile Seizures

Febrile seizures are the most common convulsive disorder of childhood. A febrile seizure is defined as a seizure associated with fever in infancy or early childhood (usually between 3 months and 5 years of age) without evidence of intracranial infection or other cause.

Febrile seizures are a benign syndrome caused by genetic factors, manifest as an age-related susceptibility to seizures, which eventually is outgrown. The problem almost always resolves without sequelae. Only a small minority will develop non-febrile seizures later. Unless seizures are exceedingly long, there is no risk of brain damage. The majority of children who have febrile seizures require no treatment.

I. **Epidemiology.** Febrile seizures occur in 2-4% of young children. The most common age of onset is in the second year of life. Higher temperature and a history of febrile seizures in a close relative are risk factors for the development of a febrile seizure.
   A. **Recurrence**
      1. After the first febrile seizure, 33% of children will experience one or more febrile seizures, and 9% of children who have febrile seizures will have 3 or more. The younger the child's age when the first febrile seizure occurs, the greater the likelihood of recurrence.
      2. Family history of febrile seizures is a risk factor for recurrence. Short duration of fever before the initial seizure and relatively lower fever at the time of the initial seizure are risk factors.
   B. **Epilepsy.** Fewer than 5% of children who have febrile seizures actually develop epilepsy. Risk factors for the development of epilepsy following febrile seizures include suspicious or abnormal development before the first seizure, family history of afebrile seizures, and complex first febrile seizure.
II. **Pathophysiology.** Most febrile illnesses associated with febrile seizures are caused by common infections (tonsillitis, upper respiratory infections, otitis media). Children of preschool age are subject to frequent infections and high fevers. These children have a relatively low seizure threshold.
III. **Clinical evaluation**
   A. Febrile seizures usually occur early in the course of a febrile illness, often as the first sign. The seizure may be of any type, but the most common is tonic-clonic. Initially there may be a cry, followed by loss of consciousness and muscular rigidity. During this tonic phase, apnea and incontinence may occur. The tonic phase is followed by the clonic phase of repetitive, rhythmic jerking movements, which is then followed by postictal lethargy or sleep.
   B. Other seizure types may be characterized by staring with stiffness or limpness or only focal stiffness or jerking. Most seizures last less than 6 minutes; 8% last longer than 15 minutes.
   C. An underlying illness that may require treatment should be sought. Symptoms of infection, medication exposure, or trauma should be assessed. The developmental level, and family history of febrile or afebrile seizures should be evaluated. A complete description of the seizure should be obtained from a witness.

D. **Physical examination**
   1. The level of consciousness, presence of meningismus, a tense or bulging fontanelle, Kernig or Brudzinski sign, and any focal abnormalities in muscle strength or tone should be sought.
   2. Encephalitis or meningitis must be excluded. A lumbar puncture (LP) is indicated if there is any suspicion of meningitis. The presence of a focus of infection (otitis media) does not preclude the possibility of meningitis.
   3. Clinical signs of meningitis may be absent in infants younger than 18 months, and the threshold for performing an LP should be low at this age. If increased intracranial pressure is present, an LP may cause fatal brain herniation, and LP is usually contraindicated.
   4. Other causes of seizures associated with fever include roseola infantum, Shigella gastroenteritis, ingestion of diphenhydramine, tricyclic antidepressants, amphetamines, cocaine, and dehydration-related electrolyte imbalances.
E. **Laboratory studies** should evaluate the source of fever. CT or MRI are seldom helpful and are not performed routinely. The electroencephalogram (EEG) is not helpful in the evaluation of febrile seizures because it is not predictive of recurrence risk of later epilepsy.

IV. **Management of febrile seizures**
   A. The child should be kept in the emergency department or physician's office for at least several hours and re-evaluated. Most children will have improved and be alert, and the child may be sent home if the cause of the fever has been diagnosed and treated. Hospital admission is necessary if the child is unstable or if meningitis remains a possibility.
   B. **Parental counseling**
      1. Parents are advised that febrile seizures do not cause brain damage, and the likelihood of developing epilepsy or recurrent non-febrile seizures is very small. There is a risk of further febrile seizures during the current or subsequent febrile illnesses.
      2. If another seizure occurs, the parent should place the child on his side or abdomen with the face downward. Nothing should be forced between the teeth. If the seizure does not stop after 10 minutes, the child should be brought to the hospital.
   C. **Control of fever** with antipyretics (acetaminophen) and sponging is recommended, but this practice has not been proven to lower the risk of recurrent febrile seizures.
   D. **Childhood immunizations.** Febrile seizures occur most commonly following a DPT immunization because pertussis provokes fever. The advantages of vaccines must be weighed against the risk of pertussis if immunization is postponed. The greatest risk for febrile seizure recurrences occurs in the 48 hours following a DPT immunization and 7 to 10 days after a measles immunization.

V. **Long-term management**
   A. Prophylaxis with diazepam or phenobarbital is not routinely necessary, but is reserved for very young children who have sustained multiple seizures associated with focal post-ictal paralysis.
   B. Diazepam may be administered orally and rectally during febrile illnesses to prevent recurrences of seizures. Oral diazepam is given in three divided doses to a total of 1 mg/kg per day when the child is ill or feverish.

References, see page 182.

Seizures and Epilepsy

Nonfebrile seizures occur at all ages. The term "seizure" designates a clinical event that represents dysfunction of the central nervous system (CNS) and may signal a serious underlying abnormality; however, more often in children the seizures result from a transient disturbance of brain function.

I. **Epidemiology and classification of seizure types**
   A. The ages of greatest risk for nonfebrile seizures are during infancy, childhood, and adolescence. The annual incidence rate from birth to 20 years of age is 0.56 per 1000. The two primary forms of epilepsy are generalized seizures and partial seizures.
   B. **Partial seizures**
      1. Partial seizures are the most common form of epilepsy in children.
      2. **Simple partial seizures (SPS)**
         a. SPS are most commonly focal, asynchronous, clonic or tonic motor movements, such as forced deviation of the head and eyes to one side.
         b. An SPS typically is short-lived, rarely persisting longer than 10 to 20 seconds, and the child remains conscious and is able to verbalize throughout the seizure. The EEG characteristically shows unilateral spikes or sharp waves in the anterior temporal region.
      3. **Complex partial seizures (CPS)**
         a. CPS initially may be similar in appearance to an SPS, but they are followed by impairment of consciousness. CPS may begin with a loss of consciousness. The average duration of a CPS is 1 to 2 minutes.
         b. **Aura** signals the onset of a seizure in 30% of children who have CPS, with the child complaining of epigastric discomfort, fear, or an unpleasant feeling.
         c. **Automatisms** are repetitive, stereotyped behaviors. These are the hallmark of CPS and occur in 50-75%. Automatisms follow the loss of consciousness, but unlike aura, the child is not aware of their presence. Automatisms may include lip smacking, chewing, repetitive swallowing, excessive salivation, picking and pulling at clothing, constant rubbing of objects, and walking and running. Automatisms are often associated with a fearful expression.
         d. During the partial seizure, the epileptiform discharge may spread from the temporal lobe to throughout the cortex, causing a generalized tonic-clonic convulsion (termed secondary generalization).
         e. During CPS, the EEG is characterized by sharp waves or spike discharges in the anterior temporal or frontal lobe, or by multifocal spikes.

International Classification of Epileptic Seizures

Partial Seizures
--Simple partial (consciousness retained)
--Complex partial (consciousness impaired)
--Partial seizure with secondary generalization

Generalized Seizures
--Absence seizures
--Myoclonic seizures
--Clonic seizures
--Tonic seizures
--Tonic-clonic seizures
--Atonic seizures

Unclassified Seizures

C. **Generalized Seizures**
1. Simple absence seizures usually have their onset at 5 to 6 years of age and are characterized by brief (5-20 sec) lapses in consciousness, speech, or motor activity. Absence seizures are not accompanied by an aura or a postictal drowsiness, but automatisms may occur, usually consisting of eye blinking or lip smacking. Hyperventilation for 3 to 4 minutes frequently induces a seizure. The EEG is characterized by 3 per second generalized spike and wave discharges.
2. Atypical absence seizures are characterized by myoclonic movements of the face and body, sometimes causing the child to fall. The EEG shows 2-2.5 per second or 3.5-4.5 per generalized spike and wave discharges.
3. Myoclonic seizures are characterized by brief, often repetitive symmetric muscle contractions with loss of normal body tone. Atonic seizures cause the child to fall because of a sudden loss of postural tone.
4. Tonic or clonic seizures are characterized by a sudden loss of consciousness and tonic-clonic, tonic, or clonic contractions. The child may develop perioral cyanosis and loss of bladder control may occur. The seizure is followed by a 30 to 60 minute period of deep sleep and postictal headache.

II. **Pathophysiology of epilepsy**
A. The etiology of most seizures in children remains unknown.
B. The acute onset of seizures may result from head injury, CNS infection (meningitis, encephalitis), cerebrovascular diseases (infarction, arteriovenous malformation, hemorrhage, venous thrombosis), toxins (lead), brain tumor, specific epilepsy syndromes, genetic/hereditary diseases (Down syndrome, tuberous sclerosis), metabolic and systemic diseases (endocrine, renal), degenerative disorders (leukodystrophy), or hereditary malformations.
C. **Hypoxic-ischemic encephalopathy** is the most common cause of seizures in the newborn, which usually are apparent within the first 24 hours. Children who have neonatal seizures following a hypoxic-ischemic insult are at significant risk to continue to have seizures.
D. **Pyridoxine dependency** may be the cause of seizures that begin shortly after birth.
E. **Metabolic encephalopathies** commonly are associated with seizures in the newborn. A urea cycle abnormality or a disorder of amino acid metabolism may cause seizures.

F. **Structural abnormalities of the brain and congenital disorders** of neuronal migration play an important role in the causation of epilepsy. Simple febrile seizures are not a cause of epilepsy.

III. Diagnosis

A. A presumptive diagnosis of epilepsy generally is made from a history of spontaneous recurrent seizures and physical examination findings. The parent usually can give a good account of the seizure and whether it was generalized or focal in onset. The child may reveal the existence of aura, which signifies a focal onset.

B. Certain seizures, such as absence or pseudoseizures, may be provoked by hyperventilation.

C. **EEG and neuroimaging studies**
   1. A routine interictal (between seizures) EEG will show an epileptiform abnormality in only 60% of patients with epilepsy. Procedures that may activate a seizure during the EEG include eye closure, hyperventilation, photic stimulation, and sleep deprivation.
   2. **MRI** is useful for excluding structural brain disorders.
   3. **Fasting blood glucose and serum calcium levels** are indicated if the history suggests hypoglycemia or hypocalcemia as a cause of the seizure.

IV. Management of nonfebrile seizures

A. **Anticonvulsant medication**
   1. Anticonvulsants are initiated following absence (typical or atypical) seizures, myoclonic seizures, and infantile spasms because the risk of recurrence is high.
   2. A single afebrile tonic-clonic seizure, particularly if it occurs on awakening, has a 75% probability of not recurring if the neurologic examination and EEG are normal and there is no family history of epilepsy. Anticonvulsants are not advised following the initial tonic-clonic seizure in these children.
   3. When two or more unprovoked afebrile seizures occur within a 6- to 12-month period, anticonvulsants usually are indicated.

Common Anticonvulsant Drugs				
Drug	Seizure Type	Oral Dose	Serum Level mcg/mL	Side Effects and Toxicities
Carbamaze-pine (Tegretol)	Partial epilepsy Tonic-clonic	Begin 10 mg/kg/d. Increase by 5 mg/kg/d every wk to 20-30 mg/kg/d in 2 or 3 divided doses	4-12	Dizziness, drowsiness, diplopia, liver, dysfunction, anemia, leukopenia
Clonazepam (Klonopin)	Myoclonic Absence	Begin 0.05 mg/kg/d. Increase by 0.05 mg/kg per wk. Maximum, 0.2 mg/kg/d in 2 or 3 divided doses	6.3-56.8	Drowsiness, irritability, drooling, behavioral abnormalities, depression

Drug	Seizure Type	Oral Dose	Serum Level mcg/mL	Side Effects and Toxicities
Ethosuximide (Zarontin)	Absence Myoclonic	Begin 10 to 20 mg/kg/d in 2 divided doses; may be increased to 50 mg/kg/d	40-160	Drowsiness, nausea, rarely blood dyscrasias
Gabapentin (Neurontin)	Partial epilepsy Tonic-clonic	Begin 300 mg/d. Increase by 300 mg/d every 3 to 5 days. Maximum 900 to 1200 mg/d in 3 equally divided doses	<2	Somnolence, dizziness. ataxia, headache, tremor, vomiting, nystagmus, fatigue.
Lamotrigine (Lamictal)	Partial epilepsy Tonic-clonic Lennox-Gastaut	Begin 2 mg/kg/d in 2 equal doses. Increase to maintenance dose of 5 to 15 mg/kg/d.	1-4	Severe skin rashes, drowsiness, headache, blurred vision.
Phenobarbital	Tonic-clonic Partial epilepsy	3 to 5 mg/kg/d in 1 or 2 divided doses	15-40	Hyperactivity, irritability, short attention span, temper tantrums, altered sleep pattern, Stevens-Johnson syndrome, depression of cognitive function.
Phenytoin (Dilantin)	Partial epilepsy Tonic-clonic	5 m 6 mg/kg/d in 2 divided doses	10-20	Hirsutism, gum hypertrophy, ataxia, skin rash, Stevens Johnson syndrome.
Primidone (Mysoline)	Tonic-clonic Partial epilepsy Myoclonic	Begin 50 mg/d in two divided doses. Gradually increase to 150 to 500 mg/d divided into 3 equal doses.	5-12	Aggressive behavior and personality changes similar to those for phenobarbital.
Sodium valproate (Depakote)	Tonic-clonic Absence Myoclonic Partial epilepsy Unclassified	Begin 10 mg/kg/d. Increase by 5 to 10 mg/kg per wk. Usual dose, 20 to 60 mg/kg/d in 2 or 3 divided doses.	50-100	Weight gain, alopecia, tremor, hepatotoxicity.

Drug	Seizure Type	Oral Dose	Serum Level mcg/mL	Side Effects and Toxicities
Vigabatrin (Sabril)	Partial epilepsy	Begin 30 to 40 mg/kg/d. Increase by 10 mg/kg per wk. Maximum, 80 to 100 mg/kg/d in 2 equal doses	1.4-14	Agitation, drowsiness, weight gain, dizziness, headache, ataxia.

- B. **Therapeutic monitoring and routine screening**
    1. Some children achieve seizure control with subtherapeutic serum drug levels (eg, carbamazepine); for others, the seizures do not come under control until serum drug levels above the usual therapeutic range are reached (eg, valproic acid).
    2. **Indications for therapeutic drug monitoring:** 1) At the initiation of therapy to ensure that the therapeutic range is achieved, 2) during times of accelerated growth, and 3) if the seizures are out of control or the child is toxic. The patient's response to treatment is more important than the serum concentration of the drug.
- C. **Surgery** is a method of treating children who have focal seizures unresponsive to anticonvulsant therapy.

References, see page 182.

Headache

Chronic or recurrent headaches occur 75% of children by 15 years. The neurogenic hypothesis proposes that cortical neuronal depression is followed by dilation and inflammation of the cranial vasculature innervated by the trigeminal nerve. Serotonin (5 hydroxytryptophan [5HT]) plays a role in this process.

I. Clinical evaluation
- A. Headaches are characterized as isolated acute, recurrent acute, chronic nonprogressive, or chronic progressive. History should exclude renal, cardiac, sinus, or dental disease or previous head trauma. A social and educational history may identify significant stresses. Past analgesic use should be determined.
- B. Physical examination should include measurement of growth parameters, head circumference, and blood pressure. The teeth should be examined and sinusitis should be sought. An arteriovenous malformation may cause an asymmetric, machinery-like cranial bruit. The child's cognitive function and emotional status should be assessed.
- C. **Papilledema.** The presence of retinal venous pulsation on funduscopy provides evidence of normal intracranial pressure. Visual acuity should be measured, and a detailed neurologic examination is essential.
- D. **Investigations.** If increased intracranial pressure or an intracranial lesion is suspected, a computed tomographic (CT) head scan should be performed. Magnetic resonance imaging (MRI) may be required to diagnose subtle vascular abnormalities or hypothalamopituitary lesions.

E. **Lumbar puncture** may be helpful if pseudotumor cerebri is suspected. However, lumbar puncture may result in herniation of the brain in patients who have obstructive hydrocephalus, an intracranial mass lesion, or cerebral edema. Neuroimaging should be performed prior to the lumbar puncture.

Physical and Neurological Examination of the Child with Headaches	
Feature	**Significance**
Growth parameters	Chronic illness may affect linear growth Hypothalamopituitary dysfunction may disturb growth
Head circumference	Increased intracranial pressure prior to fusion of the sutures may accelerate head growth
Skin	Evidence of trauma or a neurocutaneous disorder
Blood pressure	Hypertension
Neurologic examination	Signs of increased intracranial pressure Neurologic abnormality
Cranial bruits	May reflect an intracranial arteriovenous malformation

F. **Migraine**
   1. Migraines may be associated with a preceding aura, which usually involves visual phenomena. The headache is usually unilateral or bilateral, recurrent, throbbing, and associated with nausea or vomiting. Photophobia or phonophobia is common. Characteristically, the headache is relieved by sleep or by simple analgesics.
   2. A family history of migraine is obtained in up to 80% of children who have migraine. A family history of motion and travel sickness is common. Migraine episodes may be triggered by stress, lack of sleep, excitement, menstruation, or certain foods.

II. **Migraine management**
   A. **Management of acute episodes**
      1. Oral promethazine (Phenergan), 1 mg/kg up to 25 mg, often results in sleep and is generally effective. Intramuscular chlorpromazine (Compazine),1 mg/kg, can be used for severe attacks.
      2. Simple analgesics, such as acetaminophen, ibuprofen, or naproxen, may be effective.
      3. Sumatriptan (Imitrex), a selective 5-HT agonist, is an effective treatment for migraine. The subcutaneous dose of 6 mg is effective and safe in school-age children. Oral and intranasal sumatriptan spray are less effective.
      4. Intravenous dihydroergotamine mesylate (DHE) is often effective when used with metoclopramide. Metoclopramide can be given orally or intravenously prior to the DHE, which is administered over 3 minutes at a

dose of 0.5 to 1 mg. The DHE can be repeated every 8 hours. A nasal spray formulation of DHE is effective.

Treatment of Acute Migraine Episodes	
Simple analgesics	
Acetaminophen	Initial dose of 20 mg/kg PO, followed by 10 to 15 mg/kg q 4 h up to a maximum dose of 65 mg/kg per day (maximum, 3,000 mg/day)
Ibuprofen	*1 to 12 years:* 10 mg/kg PO q 4 to 6 h *More than 12 years:* 200 to 400 mg PO q 4 h; maximum dose 1,200 mg/day
Naproxen	5 mg/kg PO q 12 h; maximum dose 750 mg/day
Antiemetics	
Promethazine	Initial dose of 1 mg/kg PO (maximum, 25 mg); can be repeated at doses of 0.25 to 1 mg/kg q 4 to 6 h
Metoclopramide	0.1 to 0.2 mg/kg PO (maximum, 10 mg)
Chlorpromazine	1 mg/kg IM for severe attacks
Other Drugs	
Sumatriptan (Imitrex)	6 mg SC; may repeat in 1-2 hours; max 12 mg/day Oral: 25-50 mg PO once; may repeat in 2 hours Intranasal: 5, 10, or 20 mg in one nostril; may repeat after 2 hours
Dihydroergotamine mesylate	0.5 to 1 mg IV over 3 min in children >10 y. Can be repeated q8h. Used with metoclopramide.

B. Migraine prophylaxis. Migraine may be precipitated by stress, certain foods, lack of sleep, hormonal changes during the menstrual cycle, alcohol, and oral contraceptives. Elimination of these factors may reduce the frequency of the attacks.

Prophylactic Agents for Migraine	
Amitriptyline (Elavil)	*6-12 years:* 10 to 30 mg/day bid *Adolescents:* 10 to 50 mg/day tid
Propranolol (Inderal)	1 to 4 mg/kg per day; start at low dose and increase slowly
Riboflavin	400 mg/day as a single dose

References, see page 182.

Kawasaki Syndrome

Kawasaki syndrome (KS) is an acute, febrile, self-limited, infectious, multisystem vasculitis, which occurs in young children. Fever is often prolonged, and coronary aneurysms may lead to myocardial infarction and death.

I. **Epidemiology**
    A. Kawasaki syndrome has a peak incidence between 1 and 2 years of age. The disease is rare in children older than 8 years old, and it is uncommon before 3 months of age.
    B. Boys are affected more often than girls by a ratio of 1.5 to 1. Japanese and Korean children are at greatest risk (145 per 100,000). The rate for European children is 9 per 100,000, and the rate for African children is 20 per 100,000.

II. **Pathophysiology**
    A. Kawasaki syndrome is a multisystem vasculitis with a predilection for the coronary arteries. KS is probably caused by an infectious agent. During the first 10 days of illness, an inflammatory infiltrate appears in the coronary arteries, with pancarditis and pericarditis. Death during this phase is usually caused by an arrhythmia, although fatal heart failure may sometimes occur.
    B. **Ten to 40 days** from the onset of fever, the most common cause of death in untreated children is myocardial infarction caused by coronary aneurysms. After 40 days, healing and stenosis of the post-aneurysmal coronary artery develops.

III. **Clinical manifestations**
    A. **Abrupt onset of high but remittent fever** between 38 and 41 degrees C is characteristic of KS.
    B. **Within 2 to 5 days, the child develops other diagnostic signs of KS:** Conjunctival injection, mouth changes, an erythematous rash, changes in the hands and feet, and unilateral cervical lymphadenopathy.
    C. **Eye involvement** consists of conjunctival injection and photophobia.
    D. **The lips** are initially bright red, progressing over 3 days to swelling, cracking, and bleeding. Prominent papillae on the tongue create a strawberry appearance, and the oral cavity and pharynx is diffusely erythematous.
    E. **The skin rash** is deeply erythematous with slightly raised margins, varying in size from 2 to 3 mm papules to large plaques covering several centimeters. The rash often is urticarial and may be intensely pruritic. The rash frequently affects the face, often forming a mask-like area around the eyes, nose, and mouth. It may be distributed more prominently on the trunk or on the extremities.
    F. **Firm, indurative edema of the hands and feet** and diffuse red-purple discoloration of palms and soles develop. The edema is sharply demarcated at the wrists and around the sides of the hands and feet.
    G. **Ten to 20 days after the onset of fever**, in early convalescence, desquamation starts just under the fingernails and toenails and proceeds to involve the entire palm and sole.
    H. **Cervical lymph node involvement** occurs in 50% of patients, manifesting as sudden onset of a firm swelling on one side of the neck.

Kawasaki Syndrome: Diagnostic Criteria

I. **Fever** for ≥5 days (usually >102°F)
II. **At least four of five features**
    A. Bilateral conjunctival injection (bulbar. non-purulent)
    B. Cervical adenitis (unilateral ≥1.5 cm diameter, non-fluctuant)
    C. Rash (truncal, perineal accentuation, polymorphous but non-vesicular)
    D. Inflamed oral mucosae (fissured lips, strawberry tongue)
    E. Hand and feet inflammation (periungual peeling around 14-21 days)
III. No alternate diagnosis
IV. Fever plus 3/5 criteria are diagnostic when coronary abnormalities are present

IV. **Associated features**
    A. **Extreme irritability and emotional lability** is common.
    B. **Mild cerebrospinal fluid pleocytosis** occurs in 25%. The CSF cell count is between 50 and 150/mm^3 and is mononuclear. Protein levels are normal to slightly elevated, and glucose level is normal.
    C. **Urethritis** is present in 60% and is characterized by sterile pyuria. Red blood cells may be detected.
    D. **Severe abdominal pain** occurs in 20% in the first few days, and it may be associated with elevated amylase and lipase levels.
    E. **Liver involvement** occurs in 40%; 10% have a bilirubin level >2 mg/dL. The direct fraction is elevated.
    F. **Cardiac manifestations**
        1. Tachycardia with gallop rhythm is present in 60%, and congestive heart failure occurs in 20%. Thirty percent have a pericardial effusion, and 30% have tricuspid insufficiency.
        2. Prolongation of the PR interval and first-degree heart block are very common, but more significant arrhythmias are rare. Coronary artery aneurysms develop in 18-25%.
V. **Differential diagnosis**
    A. The differential diagnosis includes staphylococcal toxic shock syndrome, scarlatiniform erythroderma, streptococcal scarlet fever, staphylococcal scalded skin syndrome, measles, febrile viral exanthems, hypersensitivity reactions (Stevens-Johnson syndrome), and juvenile rheumatoid arthritis.
    B. KS should be considered in all young children who have a fever of unknown origin or fever and severe lymphadenopathy, rash, conjunctival injection, hand and feet changes, and mouth changes.
VI. **Laboratory findings**
    A. Erythrocyte sedimentation rate, C-reactive protein, and alpha-1-antitrypsin are elevated. White blood cell (WBC) count is elevated, with a polymorphonuclear cell predominance. Bacterial cultures should be drawn to exclude bacterial infection.
    B. Platelet counts are elevated, peaking at 650,000-2,000,000/mm^3 between days 10-20.
    C. Mild-to-moderate anemia usually is present. Bilirubin is elevated in 10%, and liver enzymes are moderately elevated in the first week in 40%. Hypoalbuminemia is common. Urinalysis shows pyuria in 60%.
VII. **Treatment of Kawasaki syndrome**
    A. **Intravenous gamma globulin.** As soon as KS is diagnosed, a baseline

echocardiogram is obtained and IVIG 2 g/kg is given in an 8- to 12-hour infusion. Heart rate and blood pressure should be monitored during the infusion.

B. Aspirin
   1. High-dose aspirin therapy is started on the same day as IVIG. The aspirin dosage is 100 mg/kg/day until a few days after defervescence or until the 14th day of illness. This is followed by a daily dose of 3 to 5 mg/kg until the ESR and platelet counts return to normal, usually after 8 weeks.
   2. Serum salicylate levels should be obtained if symptoms of toxicity (vomiting, hyperpnea, lethargy) or liver function abnormalities develop.

C. Cardiac evaluation and monitoring
   1. Serial echocardiograms should monitor the coronary arteries, valves, and ventricles.
   2. Electrocardiography is useful in the acute stage to evaluate heart block or myocarditis, QRS amplitude reduction, T wave changes, or QT interval changes.

VIII. **Prognosis.** KS usually is self-limited; however, cardiac damage may be serious. Twenty percent of all patients not treated with IVIG develop coronary artery aneurysms, appearing 7 days to 4 weeks after the onset of KS.

References, see page 182.

Juvenile Rheumatoid Arthritis

Juvenile rheumatoid arthritis (JRA) is a condition of chronic synovitis in children. The inflammation of JRA targets the synovial tissue. Affected joints are swollen, limited in motion, stiff, painful, warm, and occasionally erythematous. The etiology of JRA is unknown. Immune complex disease may perpetuate the synovitis. If synovitis persists, structures of the joint will be permanently be damaged. This destruction will be permanently damaged.

I. Clinical manifestations
   A. The American Rheumatism Association currently recognizes three subgroups: systemic-onset disease, polyarticular-onset disease, and pauciarticular-onset disease.
   B. Extraarticular manifestations of JRA include the iridocyclitis, rheumatoid nodules; fever, rash, polyserositis, hepatosplenomegaly, lymphadenopathy, anemia, leukocytosis, myocarditis, interstitial lung disease, disseminated intravascular coagulation, and amyloidosis. Growth retardation may occur with chronic JRA.
   C. Diagnosis of JRA usually requires onset of disease during childhood, presence of chronic synovitis, and exclusion of other diseases.

Objective Signs of Arthritis

Joint Swelling
--Synovial hypertrophy
--Increased amounts of synovial fluid
--Swelling of periarticular tissues
Joint Pain
--On motion
--On palpation (tenderness)
--At rest
Loss of Joint Motion
--Stiffness of joints
Joint Warmth
Joint Erythema

II. **Laboratory studies**
   A. There are no diagnostic laboratory tests for JRA. Acute phase reactants such as the erythrocyte sedimentation rate and C-reactive protein generally are elevated and present during periods of inflammation, but none of these tests is diagnostic, and a number of children have normal sedimentation rates.
   B. Standard radiographs are not diagnostic of early JRA. Joint destruction may occur in late JRA. Such late changes include narrowing of the "joint space," erosions of subchondral or juxtaarticular bone, and joint destruction. Early changes include osteoporosis, periostitis, and soft-tissue swelling.

American College of Rheumatology Criteria for Diagnosis of JRA

Diagnostic Requirements For JRA
- Documented arthritis of one or more joints for 6 weeks or longer
- Exclusion of other conditions associated with childhood arthritis
   --Other rheumatic diseases
   --Infectious diseases
   --Childhood malignancies
   --Nonrheumatic conditions of bones and joints
   --Miscellaneous conditions

III. **Therapy**
   A. Nonsteroidal anti-inflammatory drugs (NSAIDs) remain front-line agents in the treatment of JRA. NSAIDs available for use in children include salicylates, naproxen, tolmetin, ibuprofen, and indomethacin.
   B. Salicylism and salicylate hepatotoxicity may occur, and salicylates also have been associated with Reye syndrome. All of the NSAIDs may be associated with gastritis or duodenal ulcer disease. Renal and hepatic toxicity also may occur.
   C. Methotrexate is an effective agent in severe JRA, and it is recommended for children whose disease is unresponsive to NSAIDs. Doses of 10 to 15 mg/m^2 per week orally or intramuscularly are used.
   D. Disease-modifying therapies that are being tried in therapy of JRA include sulfasalazine, intravenous immunoglobulin, corticosteroid therapy, and cyclosporin. Sulfasalazine is used widely. Oral corticosteroids may be useful for severe systemic disease and iridocyclitis.

E. Physical and occupational therapy should preserve joint range of motion and muscle strength.

F. Synovectomy is of very limited usefulness. Leg length inequality, which may result from asymmetric arthritis affecting the knees, usually is transitory and can be managed by a temporary shoe lift. Soft-tissue releases can alleviate contractures, and total joint replacements may be of benefit.

References, see page 182.

Renal and Urologic Disorders

Hematuria

Hematuria occurs in about 0.5% and 1% of all children. It is defined as more than 5 to 10 RBCs per high-power microscopic field from a centrifuged midstream voided urine sample. The urine may be yellow, pink, red, brown, or smoky on gross examination. Hemoglobin and myoglobin will produce the same color changes on the dipstick as intact RBCs. A false-positive test for blood can result from the presence of ascorbic acid, sulfonamides, iron sorbitol, metronidazole, and nitrofurantoin. Therefore, each urine sample that tests positive for blood by dipstick must be examined microscopically to confirm the presence of intact RBCs.

I. **Clinical evaluation**
   A. If microscopic hematuria has been present for 1 month or more, further investigation for the cause is indicated. Vigorous exercise such as jogging or bike riding may cause hematuria. Abdominal, back, or flank pain, especially when associated with bruising, suggests child abuse. Dysuria, urinary frequency, and suprapubic pain or tenderness suggests a urinary tract infection or hypercalciuria.
   B. Abdominal pain may be associated with an abdominal mass, nephrolithiasis, or Henoch-Schönlein purpura. Aspirin, non-steroidal anti-inflammatory agents, antibiotics, methyldopa, and other drugs can cause hematuria.
   C. A history of edema, hypertension, skin rash, pallor, joint swelling or tenderness, abdominal pain, or bloody diarrhea suggests postinfectious glomerulonephritis, Henoch-Schönlein purpura, lupus nephritis, hemolytic uremic syndrome, or immunoglobulin (Ig) A nephropathy.
   D. If sore throat or pyoderma precedes the hematuria by 7 to 30 days, poststreptococcal acute glomerulonephritis must be ruled out. Hematuria with a concurrent upper respiratory infection strongly suggests IgA nephropathy. Each of these forms of glomerulonephritis usually is associated with proteinuria and RBC casts.

Evaluation of Hematuria

Patient history, family history, physical examination
Examination of urine for red blood cell casts and crystals
Screening for proteinuria with a dipstick
Examination of urine of first-degree relatives for hematuria
Urine culture
Urinary calcium/urinary creatinine; 24-hour urinary calcium excretion
Serum creatinine, C3, streptozyme titer
Renal ultrasonography
Plain abdominal film if nephrolithiasis is suspected

Differential Diagnosis of Persistent Hematuria	
Without Proteinuria	**With Proteinuria**
Urinary tract infection	Urinary tract infection
Hypercalciuria	Poststreptococcal acute glomerulonephritis
Thin basement membrane disease	IgA nephropathy
Sickle cell disease or trait	Henoch-Schönlein purpura
Renal cystic disease	Membranoproliferative glomerulonephritis
Nephrolithiasis	Lupus nephritis
Renal anatomic abnormalities	Alport syndrome Hemolytic-uremic syndrome Other forms of glomerulonephritis

E. A family history of hematuria without renal failure may be seen with thin basement membrane disease. A family history of hematuria, chronic renal failure, dialysis, or renal transplantation with bilateral deafness and ocular abnormalities suggests Alport syndrome. An audiogram is indicated for children suspected of having Alport syndrome.

F. A family history of nephrolithiasis raises the diagnostic possibility of nephrolithiasis or hypercalciuria. A family history of autosomal dominant polycystic kidney disease requires that this disease be ruled out by ultrasound. Sickle cell disease or sickle cell trait in the patient's family may suggest this diagnosis.

G. **Urinalysis.** RBCs from areas of the urinary tract other than glomeruli will be normal in size with smooth edges (eumorphic). Nonglomerular bleeding usually is associated with normal urinary protein excretion and an absence of RBC casts.

Familial Causes of Hematuria

Polycystic kidney disease
Thin basement membrane disease
Sickle cell disease or trait
Alport syndrome (hereditary nephritis with deafness)
Hypercalciuria with family history of nephrolithiasis

H. Preliminary tests should include a urine culture, blood sickle cell preparation in African-American children, urinary calcium; urinary creatinine ratio, serum creatinine; C3, and streptozyme titer. Ultrasonography of the kidneys and urinary bladder is recommended to rule out polycystic kidney disease, tumor, ureteropelvic junction obstruction, and stones.

I. The presence of proteinuria (>1+ on dipstick) strongly suggests glomerulonephritis. The diagnosis of glomerulonephritis demands microscopic inspection of the urinary sediment for the presence of RBC casts. Demonstration of RBCs that have bizarre shapes, blebs, or burrs (dysmorphic RBCs) correlates with a glomerular origin of the RBC.

J. **Proteinuria**
1. If proteinuria is present on urinalysis, urinary protein excretion should be measured by a timed 12- or 24-hour urine collection or a urine protein:urine creatinine ratio on a single voided sample. Protein excretion of less than 4 mg/m² per hour is normal; more than 40 mg/m² per hour is considered in the nephrotic range. A urine protein:urine creatinine ratio (mg/mg) greater than 0.2 is abnormal; above 1.0 is nephrotic range proteinuria.
2. A complete blood count, C3, C4, antistreptolysin-O titer, streptozyme titer, serum electrolytes, blood urea nitrogen, serum creatinine, serum albumin, test for lupus erythematosus, hepatitis B screen, and antinuclear cytoplasmic antibody titer are indicated to clarify the type of glomerulonephritis. A screening urinalysis on first-degree family members is also important. When confirmatory serologic tests are nondiagnostic, a renal biopsy usually is indicated.

Renal Structural Abnormalities Associated with Hematuria

Polycystic kidney disease
Ureteropelvic junction obstruction
Vesicoureteral reflux
Renal or bladder stones, diverticulae or tumors
Renal arteriovenous fistula
Foreign bodies

References, see page 182.

Fluids and Electrolytes

Disorders affecting the body fluids and electrolytes are treated by supplying maintenance requirements, correcting volume and electrolyte deficits, and by replacing ongoing abnormal losses.

I. **Dehydration**
A. **Maintenance fluid and electrolytes**
1. Sensible losses, primarily urinary, account for approximately 50% of daily fluid requirements. Caloric requirements for growth can be estimated as equivalent on a kcal-for-mL basis to water requirements.
2. Factors that increase the requirements for calories and water are fever (10% for each degree), physical activity, ongoing gastrointestinal losses, hyperventilation, and hypermetabolic states. Anuria, oliguria, and congestive heart failure may reduce the requirements for water.

Maintenance Requirements for Fluid and Electrolytes			
Body Weight	**0 to 10 kg**	**10 to 20 kg**	**>20 kg**
Water Volume	100 mL/kg	1000 mL + 50 mL/kg for each kg >10 kg	1500 mL + 20 mL/kg for each kg >20 kg
Sodium	3 mEq/kg	3 mEq/kg	3 mEq/kg
Potassium	2 mEq/kg	2 mEq/kg	2 mEq/kg
Chloride	5 mEq/kg	5 mEq/kg	5 mEq/kg

3. Abnormal losses, such as those arising from nasogastric aspiration, prolonged diarrhea or burns, should be measured, and replaced on a volume for volume basis.
B. **Estimation of deficit**
 1. Estimation of volume depletion should assess fever, vomiting, diarrhea, and urine output. Recent feeding, including type and volume of food and drink, and weight change should be determined.

Estimation of Dehydration			
Degree of Dehydration	**Mild**	**Moderate**	**Severe**
Weight Loss--Infants	5%	10%	15%
Weight Loss--Children	3-4%	6-8%	10%
Pulse	Normal	Slightly increased	Very increased
Blood Pressure	Normal	Normal to orthostatic, >10 mm Hg change	Orthostatic to shock
Behavior	Normal	Irritable	Hyperirritable to lethargic
Thirst	Slight	Moderate	Intense
Mucous Membranes	Normal	Dry	Parched
Tears	Present	Decreased	Absent tears, sunken eyes
Anterior Fontanelle	Normal	Normal to sunken	Sunken
External Jugular Vein	Visible when supine	Not visible except with supraclavicular pressure	Not visible even with supraclavicular pressure

Degree of Dehydration	Mild	Moderate	Severe
Skin	Capillary refill <2 sec	Delayed capillary refill, 2-4 sec (decreased turgor)	Very delayed capillary refill (>4 sec), tenting; cool, acrocyanotic, or mottled skin
Urine Specific Gravity (SG)	>1.020	>1.020; oliguria	Oliguria or anuria

2. The percent dehydration is used to calculate the milliliters of body water deficit per kilogram of body weight.

C. Isonatremic dehydration
1. The most common cause of dehydration in infants is diarrhea. Children who have a brief illness and anorexia usually present with isotonic dehydration.

2. Oral rehydration
   a. Moderate volume depletion should be treated with oral fluids. The majority of patients who have gastroenteritis can be treated with oral rehydration therapy.
   b. Small aliquots of oral hydration solution (Ricelyte, Pedialyte, Resol, Rehydralyte) are given as tolerated to provide 50 mL/kg over 4 hours in mild dehydration, and up to 100 mL/kg over 6 hours in moderate dehydration. Once rehydration is accomplished, maintenance fluid is given at 100 mL/kg per day. Clear-liquid beverages, such as broths, juices, sodas, and tea, are inappropriate for the treatment of dehydration.

3. Parenteral rehydration
   a. Parenteral fluids should be given for severe volume depletion, altered states of consciousness, intractable vomiting, and abdominal distention or ileus.
   b. The first phase of treatment rapidly expands the vascular volume. Intravenous normal saline or Ringers lactate (10-20 mL/kg) should be given over 1 hour.
   c. The next phase of treatment is aimed at correcting the deficit, providing maintenance, and replacing ongoing abnormal losses. In severe depletion, half of the calculated deficit is given over the first 8 hours and the second half over the next 16 hours; maintenance needs are provided at a steady rate. Five percent glucose should be used as the stock solution and NaCl is added according to the estimated need. Children who have isonatremic dehydration require 8 to 10 mEq of Na^+ per kg of body weight for repletion of deficit and 3 mEq/kg per day for maintenance. This Na^+ is given in a volume consisting of the calculated maintenance for water and the estimated water deficit. Once urine flow occurs, KCl is added at a concentration of 20 mEq/L.

D. Hyponatremia and hyponatremic dehydration
1. The signs and symptoms of hyponatremia correlate with the rapidity and extent of the fall in serum Na^+ concentration. Symptoms include apathy, nausea, vomiting, cramps, weakness, headache, seizures, and coma.
2. If the correction of fluid and electrolyte losses is excessively rapid, the brain may sustain injury caused by dehydration. In severe hyponatremia, plasma

Na$^+$ concentration should be corrected at no more than 10-12 mEq/L/day.

3. **Differential diagnosis of hyponatremia**

   a. **Hypovolemia**

      (1) The most frequent cause of hypovolemic hyponatremia is viral gastroenteritis with vomiting and diarrhea. Other causes of hypovolemic hyponatremia include percutaneous losses or third space sequestration of fluid (ascites, burns, peritonitis).

      (2) Renal sodium loss (urinary Na$^+$ >20 mEq/L) may be caused by diuretics, salt-wasting nephropathy, proximal renal tubular acidosis, and lack of or resistance to mineralocorticoid.

   b. **Euvolemia.** The most common cause of euvolemic hyponatremia is the syndrome of inappropriate antidiuretic hormone secretion, which is caused by water retention (urinary Na$^+$ is usually >20 mEq/L). Causes include tumors, pulmonary disorders, CNS infection, and certain drugs. Euvolemic hyponatremia may also occur in infants fed excessively diluted infant formula.

   c. **Hypervolemia.** Hypervolemic hyponatremia, associated with edema, may result from water retention and excess Na$^+$, as in nephrosis, congestive heart failure, cirrhosis, or renal failure.

4. **Management of hyponatremia**

   a. Hypovolemic patients who have hyponatremia first require volume repletion with normal saline, then a solution containing salt is given to correct the Na$^+$ deficit (10 to 12 mEq/kg of body weight or 15 mEq/kg in severe hyponatremia) and to provide the Na$^+$ maintenance needs (3 mEq/kg per day) in a 5% dextrose solution.

   b. For a serum Na$^+$ concentration of 120 to 130 mEq/L, this amount should be given over a 24-hour period. For a serum Na$^+$ concentration <120 mEq/L, the rehydration should be spread out over several days at a rate of 10 mEq/day.

   c. **Symptomatic hyponatremia** (headache, lethargy, disorientation) requires urgent therapy to prevent seizures or coma.

      (1) Hypertonic saline (3% saline solution), with or without a loop diuretic and water restriction, should be used to raise the serum Na$^+$ by 1 to 2 mEq/L per hour or halfway toward normal during the first 8 hours.

      (2) A correction using 3% saline over 4 hours can be calculated according to the following formula:

$$\text{Sodium deficit in mEq} = \frac{(125 - \text{observed [Na}^+\text{])}}{\text{kg} \times 0.6} \times \text{body weight in}$$

E. **Hypernatremia and hypernatremic dehydration**

   1. The hypernatremic patient is usually also dehydrated. Total body Na$^+$ most commonly is decreased. Affected patients frequently exhibit lethargy or confusion, muscle twitching, hyperreflexia, or convulsions. Fever is common, and the skin may feel thickened or doughy.

   2. **Differential Diagnosis**

      a. Diarrhea, which usually results in isonatremic or hyponatremic dehydration, may cause hypernatremia in the presence of persistent fever, anorexia, vomiting, and decreased fluid intake.

      b. Other causes of hypernatremia include water and Na$^+$ deficit from skin losses or renal losses, and water losses from central or nephrogenic diabetes insipidus (DI) or drugs (lithium, cyclophosphamide).

3. **Management**
   a. Initial therapy requires administration of normal saline or Ringers lactate to restore circulating plasma volume. Hypovolemic patients who have hypernatremia require a hypotonic solution containing salt to restore the Na^+ deficit (2-5 mEq/kg of body weight) and to provide the Na^+ maintenance (3 mEq/kg of Na^+) in a solution containing 20-40 mmol/L of KCl and 5% glucose.
   b. For a serum Na^+ concentration of 150-160 mEq/L, this volume should be given over 24-hours. An elevated serum Na^+ concentration should be corrected by no more than 10 mEq/L per day.
   c. For a serum Na^+ concentration >160 mEq/L, the rehydration should be spread out over several days to lower the Na^+ concentration to 150 mEq/L by 10 mEq/day.

II. Potassium disorders
A. Abnormalities of serum K^+ are potentially life-threatening because of effects on cardiac function.

B. **Hypokalemia**
   1. Hypokalemia (serum K^+ concentration <3 mEq/L) is most frequently caused by gastrointestinal K^+ losses or renal losses (nasogastric suction, protracted vomiting, diuretics, renal tubular disease). Manifestations of hypokalemia include arrhythmias, neuromuscular excitability (hyporeflexia or paralysis, decreased peristalsis, ileus), and rhabdomyolysis.
   2. Intracellular K^+ concentration can be estimated from the electrocardiogram, which may reveal flattened T waves, shortened P-R interval and QRS complex, and eventually U waves.
   3. **Management**
      a. In the presence of cardiac arrhythmias, extreme muscle weakness, or respiratory distress, patients should receive KCl intravenously with cardiac monitoring. Once the serum K^+ is stabilized, oral administration is preferable.
      b. If the patient is likely to be hypophosphatemic, a phosphate salt should be used. In metabolic alkalosis, KCl should be used; in renal tubular acidosis, a citrate salt should be used.

C. **Hyperkalemia**
   1. The most common cause of hyperkalemia (K^+ >5.5 mEq/L) is "pseudohyperkalemia" from hemolysis of the blood sample. This cause should be excluded by repeating the measurement on a free-flowing venous sample. Children may display hyperkalemia in metabolic acidosis, tissue catabolism, renal failure, volume depletion, or hypoaldosteronism.
   2. In salt-losing congenital adrenal hyperplasia, due to complete deficiency of the enzyme 21-hydroxylase, the symptoms in affected male infants appear in the first weeks of life and include dehydration and failure to thrive together with low serum Na^+ and high K^+ concentrations. Affected female infants usually are diagnosed at birth because of ambiguous genitalia. Nonsteroidal anti-inflammatory agents may also induce hyperkalemia.
   3. Manifestations of hyperkalemia include cardiac arrhythmias, paresthesias, muscle weakness, and paralysis.
   4. The electrocardiogram demonstrates narrow, peaked T waves and shortened QT intervals at K^+ concentrations >6 mEq/L and depressed ST segment and widened QRS complex at K^+ concentrations >8 mEq/L.
   5. **Management**
      a. Emergent therapy to reverse potentially life-threatening hyperkalemia consists of intravenous calcium. The onset of action is rapid; however,

the duration is less than 30 minutes.

    b. Emergent administration of glucose will cause K^+ to redistribute to the intracellular space. Glucose, 0.5 gm/kg, can be given over 30-60 minutes when EKG changes are present.

    c. Sodium polystyrene sulfonate (Kayexalate) (1 gm/kg) can be given by high rectal enema or orally. Severe hyperkalemia is treated with hemodialysis.

III. Acid-base disorders

  A. The pH of the body fluids normally is between 7.35 and 7.45.

  B. **Metabolic acidosis**

    1. Acidosis results from the addition of acid or the removal of alkali from body fluids, and it causes a compensatory increase in ventilation (respiratory alkalosis) and a fall in Pco_2 Manifestations of acidosis include depressed myocardial contractility, arrhythmias, hypotension, and pulmonary edema.

    2. **Diagnosis**

      a. Addition of a fixed acid to the extracellular fluid causes the formation of unmeasured anions. These unmeasured anions are referred to as the anion gap, which can be estimated as:

$$\text{Anion gap} = Na^+ - (Cl + HCO_3^-) = 10\text{-}12 \text{ mEq/L}$$

    3. **Differential diagnosis**

      a. **Normal anion gap (hyperchloremic) acidosis**

        (1) This disorder occurs when HCO_3^- is lost from the body, either through the gastrointestinal tract or the kidneys. Diarrheal fluid is high in HCO_3^-, high in K^+, and low in Cl^-. Thus, diarrhea causes hypokalemia and hyperchloremic acidosis.

        (2) Failure to excrete acid occurs in mild chronic renal insufficiency and RTA.

      b. **Increased anion gap acidosis** may be caused by diabetic ketoacidosis, lactic acidosis, ingestion of toxins (aspirin, ethylene glycol), and renal failure.

    4. **Treatment of acidosis**

      a. Bicarbonate should be given when plasma HCO_3^- is <5 mmol/L. Bicarbonate should be added to a hypotonic solution and given as a continuous infusion over 1 hour. The amount to infuse is calculated with the following formula:

$$\text{Amount to infuse in mEq} = \text{weight in kg } (15 - \text{observed } [HCO_3^-]) \times 0.5$$

      b. With severe watery diarrhea, resulting in moderate-to-severe metabolic acidosis, volume replacement is the primary mode of therapy.

  C. **Metabolic alkalosis**

    1. Alkalosis results from a gain of base or a loss of acid. The common clinical manifestations are lethargy, confusion, neuromuscular irritability, arrhythmias, and seizures.

    2. **Differential diagnosis**

      a. Causes of metabolic alkalosis include alkali administration, vomiting, and nasogastric aspiration. In patients with GI loss of acid from vomiting, urinary Cl^- concentration is usually below 20 mEq/L.

      b. Cushing syndrome, Bartter syndrome or primary aldosteronism may cause metabolic alkalosis.

3. **Treatment**
   a. Therapy consists of identifying and treating the underlying pathology.
   b. In mild-to-moderate alkalosis, provision of Cl⁻ will allow the kidney to excrete the excess base. In severe alkalosis, hydrochloric acid administration may be necessary.

D. **Respiratory acidosis**
   1. Respiratory acidosis is induced by an increase in Pco_2 which lowers plasma pH. Causes of respiratory acidosis include airway obstruction, and pulmonary disorders.
   2. Treatment consists of mechanical ventilation and correction of the underlying disorder.

E. **Respiratory alkalosis**
   1. Respiratory alkalosis is caused by a decrease in Pco_2, secondary to hyperventilation, resulting in dizziness, confusion, and seizures.
   2. Causes of respiratory alkalosis include hyperventilation caused by CNS disorders and panic disorder. Treatment involves correcting the underlying disorder. Rebreathing into a bag may decrease the severity of symptoms.

References, see page 182.

Vesicoureteral Reflux

Vesicoureteral reflux is defined as the retrograde flow of urine from the bladder into the ureter and collecting system. Children who have a urinary tract infection (UTI) have a 45% incidence of vesicoureteral reflux. The incidence increases with decreasing age, and 65% of patients are females. In a male who has a UTI, the risk of reflux is 30%. Vesicoureteral reflux may cause renal parenchymal injury, including segmental scarring, global renal atrophy, and renal growth failure.

I. **Diagnosis**
   A. **Radiologic evaluation** for vesicoureteral reflux should be undertaken when a urinary tract infection occurs in one of the following patients:
      1. UTI in a male
      2. UTI in an infant (under two years of age)
      3. Pyelonephritis in a female
      4. Recurrent UTI in a female
   B. Radiologic evaluation of the child with a urinary tract infection consists of a renal ultrasound and a voiding cystourethrogram (VCUG). If the child is not toxic, the VCUG and renal ultrasound should be done three weeks after initiation of antibiotics for UTI. However, if the child is toxic or hospitalized, the ultrasound should be done promptly in order to exclude the presence of an obstructive uropathy, which requires prompt urological intervention.
   C. **Grading of vesicoureteral reflux**
      1. **Grade I reflux** is defined as retrograde urine flow into a non-dilated ureter.
      2. **Grade II reflux** refers to the filling of a non-dilated ureter and a non-dilated renal pelvis.
      3. **Grade III reflux** consists of dilatation of the collecting system, but the fornices remain sharp.
      4. **Grade IV reflux** consists of blunted fornices.
      5. **Grade V reflux** is defined as massive dilatation and tortuosity of the collecting system.

II. Medical management

A. Most cases of vesicoureteral reflux are managed nonoperatively with attention to perineal hygiene, normalization of bowel and voiding habits, and prophylactic antibiotics.

B. Diaper rashes and chemical irritants such as bubble bath should be discouraged because they predispose to UTIs. Children should avoid harsh soaps, shampoos, and tub baths. If constipation is a problem, stool softeners and scheduled defecation programs are effective.

C. Prophylactic antibiotics

   1. Trimethoprim/sulfamethoxazole is the most commonly used drug, given in a dose of 2mg/kg of trimethoprim plus 10mg/kg of sulfamethoxazole, orally once a day before bedtime. Adverse reactions may include Stevens Johnson syndrome, allergies, and blood dyscrasias. For the newborn, penicillin or ampicillin are preferred for prophylaxis.

   2. Suppression continues until the reflux resolves spontaneously or until surgery is performed.

D. Patient monitoring

   1. Urine cultures are obtained for 3 months after any UTI. Thereafter, a urine culture is obtained every other month for 6 months. If the urine remains sterile, surveillance cultures are then obtained every 3 months.

   2. Repeat imaging is obtained every 6-12 months. Follow-up can be done with a nuclear cystogram. Patients who have minimal or no scarring may only need an ultrasound.

E. Surgical management

   1. Absolute indications for ureteral reimplantation include progressive renal injury or breakthrough infections, despite urinary suppression.

   2. Patients who have grade V vesicoureteral reflux should be managed by ureteral reimplantation. Relative indications for surgery include grade IV reflux and failure of reflux to resolve following 4 years of therapy.

References

References for this book can be obtained at www.ccspublishing.com/ccs.

Index

Titles from Current Clinical Strategies Publishing

In All Medical Bookstores Worldwide

Family Medicine, 2000 Edition
Outpatient Medicine, 2001 Edition
History and Physical Examination, 2001-2002 Edition
Medicine, 2001 Edition
Pediatrics 5-Minute Reviews, 2001-2002 Edition
Anesthesiology, 1999-2000 Edition
Handbook of Psychiatric Drugs, 2001-2002 Edition
Gynecology and Obstetrics, 1999-2000 Edition
Manual of HIV/AIDS Therapy, 2001 Edition
Practice Parameters in Medicine and Primary Care, 1999-2000
    Edition
Surgery, 1999-2000 Edition
Pediatric Drug Reference, 2000 Edition
Critical Care Medicine, 2000 Edition
Psychiatry, 1999-2000 Edition
Pediatrics, 2000 Edition
Physicians' Drug Manual, 2001 Edition
Pediatric History and Physical Examination, Fourth Edition

CD-ROM and Softcover Book

Clinical Guidelines in Fam. Prac.
Up Hold & Graham - 4th Ed.

Tb Rx

Isoniazid tabs 300mg QD
Rifampin caps 300mg QD
Pyrazinamide tabs 500mg QD
B₆ tabs 50mg QD

Isoniazid & Rifampin
    daily x 9 months

Pyrazinamide & Ethambutal
    & Isoniazid daily x 2 months
